A GREAT AND
GROWING
EVIL

THE ROYAL COLLEGE OF PHYSICIANS

A GREAT AND GROWING EVIL

The medical consequences
of alcohol abuse

TAVISTOCK: LONDON AND NEW YORK

First published in 1987
by Tavistock Publications Ltd
11 New Fetter Lane, London EC4P 4EE
Reprinted 1987

Published in the USA by
Tavistock Publications
in association with Methuen, Inc.
29 West 35th Street, New York NY 10001

Printed in Great Britain by
Richard Clay (The Chaucer Press) Ltd
Bungay, Suffolk

British Library Cataloguing in Publication Data
Royal College of Physicians of London
A great and growing evil? : the medical
consequences of alcohol abuse.
1. Alcohol—Physiological effect
I. Title
615'.7828   QP801.A3
ISBN 0–422–61140–9
ISBN 0–422–61150–6 Pbk

Library of Congress Cataloging in Publication Data
Royal College of Physicians of London.
A Great and Growing Evil?
(Social Science Paperbacks: 356)
Includes bibliographies and index.
Prepared by the working party on alcohol.
1. Alcoholism.   2. Alcohol—Physiological effect.
3. Alcoholism—Great Britain. I. Royal
College of Physicians of London. Working Party on
Alcohol.   *II. Title.   III. Series. (DNLM: 1. Alcoholism—*
complications. WM 274 R8873G)
RC565.R587 1987 616.86'1 86–30176
ISBN 0–422–61140–9
ISBN 0–422–61150–6 (Pbk.)

CONTENTS

MEMBERSHIP OF THE WORKING PARTY ON ALCOHOL

Sir Raymond Hoffenberg   *Chairman*
Dr R. F. Mahler   *Honorary Secretary*

Dr D. J. P. Barker
Dr D. G. Beevers
Dr J. C. Catford
Dr A. M. Dawson
Dr D. Hull
Dr M. A. McDonald
Dr Marsha Y. Morgan
Dr Celia M. Oakley
Dr A. Paton
Dr D. A. Pyke   *Registrar of the College*
Dr R. Smith
Dr P. K. Thomas
Dr A. D. Thomson
Mr G. M. G. Tibbs   *Secretary of the College*

ACKNOWLEDGEMENTS

The Royal College of Physicians acknowledges with thanks a donation from Dalgety plc towards the costs incurred in the production of the report on the medical consequences of alcohol abuse.

SUMMARY OF RECOMMENDATIONS FOR REDUCING ALCOHOL ABUSE

Sensible limits of drinking

Men

Not more than 21 units (see *Figure 1*, p.5) a week including 2 or 3 days without any alcohol.

Women

Not more than 14 units a week including 2 or 3 days without any alcohol.

What doctors must do

- Improve early detection of people at risk by taking a careful drinking history.
- Determine the extent of drinking by people at work and by patients attending their practices and clinics.
- Educate the public to drink within 'safe' limits.
- Give better instruction to medical students and doctors-in-training on the problems arising from alcohol abuse.

What government can do

- Help to reduce the nation's overall consumption to 'safe' limits by price control and by not liberalizing licensing laws further.
- Control the nature and extent of alcohol advertisements.
- Adopt a much tougher drinking-and-driving policy.
- Support research and education leading to detection and prevention of alcohol problems.
- Set up a single government body to coordinate all aspects of alcohol use and abuse.

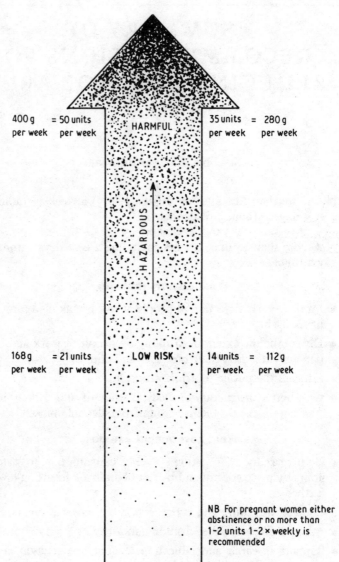

MEN   WOMEN

400 g   = 50 units   35 units   =   280 g
per week   per week   per week   per week

HARMFUL

HAZARDOUS

168 g   = 21 units   14 units   =   112 g
per week   per week   per week   per week

LOW RISK

NB For pregnant women either
abstinence or no more than
1–2 units 1–2 × weekly is
recommended

1

THE EXTENT OF
THE PROBLEM

'Alcohol misuse is a social problem with medical complications.'
(Sir Desmond Pond, Former Chief Scientist, DHSS)

This is not the first time that the Royal College of Physicians has felt
it necessary to draw public attention to the harm caused by the
immoderate use of alcohol. In 1726 it made a submission to the
House of Commons on 'a great and growing evil' later to be
compellingly portrayed by Hogarth in his engraving of Gin Lane.

'We the President and College or Commonalty of the Faculty of
Physicians in London, who are appointed by the Laws of this
Kingdom to take care of the health of his Majesties Subjects in
London and within seven miles circuit of the same, do think it
our Duty most humbly to represent that we have with concern,
observed, for some years past, the fatal effects of the frequent use
of several sorts of distilled Spirituous Liquors upon great
numbers of both Sexes, rend(e)ring them diseased, not fit for
business, poor, a burthen to themselves and neighbours and too
often the cause of weak, feeble and distempered children, who
must be, instead of an advantage and strength, a charge to their
country. We crave leave further most humbly to represent, that
this Custom doth every year increase, notwithstanding our
repeated advices to the contrary.
We therefore most humbly submit to the Consideration of
Parliament, so great and growing an evil.'
(Minutes of a meeting of the Royal College of Physicians, 1726)

Now, 260 years later, we have once again been led to write a report
because of the increasing number of patients we see who are
damaged by alcohol. About one in five of all men admitted to
medical wards has a problem related to alcohol abuse,[1–9] and a recent

study of medical outpatients has shown that 10–20 per cent drink more than 80 g (10 units) of alcohol a day[4] – an amount that may result in physical damage. Estimates of the number of alcohol-dependent people in England and Wales vary between 70,000 and 240,000, and of the number of problem drinkers between 0.5 and 1.3 million.[8] Many of these individuals suffer physical, psychological, social, and occupational harm.

The main aim of this report is to illustrate and draw attention to the fact that alcohol produces wide-ranging physical harm and that no system in the body is immune from its effects.

Our report is aimed not only at doctors, but also at the general public, health authorities, members of Parliament, and the Government, because we believe that there is considerable ignorance among all these groups[10–12] as to the depth and breadth of the problems associated with the use and misuse of alcohol.[12–20] It is important that the public and the Government understand the importance of alcohol in causing wide-ranging harm because the prevention of this cannot come from health professions alone. Alcohol problems are more easily prevented than treated, but if problems are to be prevented then individuals and controlling bodies must be provided with the necessary information upon which to make decisions and formulate plans.

Our sister colleges, the Royal College of Psychiatrists and the Royal College of General Practitioners,[21,22] have also prepared reports to express their concern about the alcohol-related problems seen increasingly by their members. As physicians, we have chosen to concentrate on the physical problems associated with alcohol abuse. They are listed in *Table 1* and elaborated in the relevant sections of this report.

We want to draw attention to the fact that alcohol-related disease is not confined to a relatively small number of individuals with 'skid row' problems of social and physical disintegration. Alcohol can cause medical illness when consumed at much lower levels than previously thought. Regular consumption of 60 g (7.5 units) of alcohol a day, equivalent to a daily intake of about four pints of beer, is associated with an increasing risk of sickness from high blood pressure, strokes, liver disease, infertility, and diseases of the nervous system. In women, half that amount puts them at increasing risk of developing illnesses.

Many individuals who are substantially harming themselves with alcohol may show no physical, social, or emotional side effects in the early stages. It is usually only by careful questioning about alcohol

Table 1 *Summary of physical health hazards associated with alcohol abuse*

Nervous system
Acute intoxication; 'black-outs'
Persistent brain damage:
  Wernicke's encephalopathy
  Korsakoff's syndrome
  cerebellar degeneration
  dementia
Cerebrovascular disease:
  strokes, especially in young people
  subarachnoid haemorrhage
  subdural haematoma after head injury
Withdrawal symptoms:
  tremor, hallucinations, fits
Nerve and muscle damage:
  weakness, paralysis, burning sensations in hands and feet

Liver
Infiltration of liver with fat
Alcoholic hepatitis
Cirrhosis and eventual liver failure
Liver cancer

Gastrointestinal system
Reflux of acid into the oesophagus
Tearing and occasionally rupture of the oesophagus
Cancer of the oesophagus
Gastritis
Aggravation and impaired healing of peptic ulcers
Diarrhoea and impaired absorption of food
Chronic inflammation of the pancreas leading in some to diabetes and
  malabsorption of food

Nutrition
Malnutrition from reduced intake of food, toxic effects of alcohol on
  intestine, and impaired metabolism, leading to weight loss
Obesity, particularly in early stages of heavy drinking

Heart and circulatory system
Abnormal rhythms
High blood pressure
Chronic heart muscle damage leading to heart failure

Respiratory system
Fractured ribs
Pneumonia from inhalation of vomit

Table 1 (*cont.*)

Endocrine system
Overproduction of cortisol leading to obesity, acne, increased facial hair, and high blood pressure
Condition mimicking over-activity of the thyroid with loss of weight, anxiety, palpitations, sweating, and tremor
Severe fall in blood sugar, sometimes leading to coma
Intense facial flushing in many diabetics taking the anti-diabetic drug chlorpropamide

Reproductive system
In men, loss of libido, reduced potency, shrinkage in size of testes and penis, reduced or absent sperm formation and so infertility, and loss of sexual hair
In women, sexual difficulties, menstrual irregularities, and shrinkage of breasts and external genitalia

Occupation and accidents
Impaired work performance and decision making
Increased risk and severity of accidents

The fetus, the child, and the family
Damage to the fetus and the fetal alcohol syndrome
Acute intoxication in young children:
    hypothermia, low blood sugar levels, depressed respiration
Effect on physical development and behaviour of the child through heavy drinking by parents

Interaction of alcohol with medicinal substances
Increased likelihood of unwanted effects of drugs
Reduced effectiveness of medicines

---

intake and by measuring several biochemical and haematological markers that it is possible to identify that a disease is alcohol-related.

In this report we shall draw attention to the many and varied ways in which alcohol can harm the body; and we will also discuss the strengths and weaknesses of the evidence that associates them.

Definitions

Throughout this report we use the term alcohol to refer solely to ethanol. There are many other natural and synthetic alcohols, but almost all are either highly toxic or undrinkable, or both.

A 'standard' drink is referred to in this report as 'a unit' and contains 8 g of pure alcohol. *Figure 1* shows the standard public house measures, each of which provides one unit of alcohol.

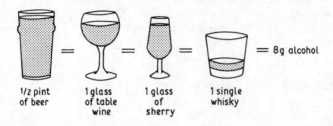

| 1/2 pint of beer | 1 glass of table wine | 1 glass of sherry | 1 single whisky | = 8g alcohol |

Figure 1 One unit, or 8 g, of alcohol.

A can of beer or lager (450 ml) contains nearly 1.5 units (12 g), a bottle of wine about 7 (56 g), a bottle of sherry or port 15 (120 g), and a standard bottle of spirits and most liqueurs 30 units (230–250 g). These figures are only approximate because there is wide variation in the amount of alcohol in different alcoholic drinks (*Table 2*) and the size of a measure also varies from place to place throughout Britain.

Table 3 gives definitions of 'social drinker', 'heavy drinker', 'problem drinker', and 'dependent drinker'. We must emphasize, however, that these divisions are arbitrary: social drinkers merge into heavy drinkers; some people who drink a little experience greater problems than some who drink more; and an individual who is drinking 'heavily' today may be 'dependent' tomorrow and vice versa. Terms like 'alcoholic' and 'alcoholism', though widely used, are impossible to define and we do not use them in this report because they also carry with them the mistaken idea that the condition is irreversible and untreatable.

Although it is true that the later stages have a poor outlook, recovery or arrest of the damage is possible in many cases without medical treatment.[23] It is also incorrect to think that only 'alcoholics' suffer problems through excessive drinking. Likewise, the idea that only a minority of the population is genetically and physically capable of becoming dependent on alcohol is misleading. Genetic factors may be important but, as yet, it is impossible to identify individuals doomed to alcohol dependence or those who are immune.

A man who regularly drinks more than an average of 8 units (64 g)

Table 2 *Alcohol content of various beverages*

beverage	grams of alcohol	units of alcohol
beers and lagers		
ordinary strength	8 g/½ pint	1
beer or lager	12 g/can	1.5
(3% alcohol)	16 g/pint	2
export beer	16 g/can	2
(4% alcohol)	20 g/pint	2.5
strong beer	16 g/½ pint	2
or lager	24 g/can	3
(5.5% alcohol)	32 g/pint	4
extra strength	20 g/½ pint	2.5
beer or lager	32 g/can	4
(7% alcohol)	40 g/pint	5
ciders		
average cider	12 g/½ pint	1.5
(4% alcohol)	24 g/pint	3
strong cider	16 g/½ pint	2
(6% alcohol)	32 g/pint	4
	64 g/quart bottle	8
spirits		
whisky 70 proof	8 g/single measure	
(32% alcohol)	in England and Wales	1
or		
brandy 70 proof	12 g/single measure	
(32% alcohol)	in Scotland and N. Ireland	1.5
or		
whisky 70 proof	240g/bottle	30
(32% alcohol)		
or		
vodka 70 proof	240 g/bottle	30
(32% alcohol)		
or		
gin 70 proof	240 g/bottle	30
(32% alcohol)		
table wines		
(8–10% alcohol)	8 g/standard glass	1
	56 g/bottle	7
	100 g/litre bottle	12.5
fortified wine		
sherry		
port	8 g/standard measure	1
Vermouth	120 g/bottle	15
(13–16% alcohol)		
liqueurs		
(15–30% alcohol)	8 g/small measure	1
	100–240 g/bottle	12.5–30

Table 3 *Definitions of different kinds of drinkers*

Social drinker

Someone who drinks usually not more than 2–3 units of alcohol a day and does not become intoxicated, is not likely to harm him- or herself or family through drinking. The amount that can be drunk without harm varies widely between individuals, but greater amounts than this are associated with increasing risk of harm.

Heavy drinker

Someone who regularly drinks more than 6 units of alcohol a day but without apparent immediate harm.

Problem drinker

Someone who experiences physical, psychological, social, family, occupational, financial, or legal problems attributable to drinking.

Dependent drinker

Someone who has a compulsion to drink; takes roughly the same amount each day; has increased tolerance to alcohol in the early stages and reduced tolerance later; suffers withdrawal symptoms if alcohol is stopped which are relieved by consuming more; in whom drinking takes precedence over other activities and who tends to resume drinking after a period of abstinence.

---

alcohol a day and a woman who regularly drinks more than an average of 5 units (40 g) alcohol a day stands a high chance of damage. Anyone who becomes intoxicated is liable to a wide range of problems associated specifically with drunkenness, especially accidents and assault.

Benefits and Risks

Doctors are not prohibitionists. However, because the amount of alcohol consumed by a population and the amount of damage caused are closely related, alcohol problems will only diminish when less alcohol is consumed and suitable drinking limits are observed (see p. 108). Moreover, what the nation spends on alcohol it cannot spend on other things that could improve its health and well-being.

Social and Economic Problems

The British spend more on alcohol than they do on clothes, cars, hospitals, schools, or universities. In 1981 this came to over £11,000 m, representing 7.5 per cent of consumer expenditure.[24]

Alcohol is usually available at christenings, weddings, and funerals, at the launching of ships and at office parties. The sense of well-being associated with a blood alcohol concentration of 20 mg/100 ml (after drinking 1 unit) is clearly greatly appreciated, as too, is the mild disinhibition experienced when the blood level reaches 40 mg/100 ml (after drinking 2 units). The individual and social value of alcohol may be hard to define, and the protective effect of a little alcohol against heart disease is not proven (see p. 27), but the economic benefits to the Government from alcohol revenue are more easily measured. The Government collected £5,825 million in excise duty and value-added tax from the sale of alcohol in 1983–84.[25] Exports of alcohol are worth more than £1,000 million a year, giving, at the moment, a positive balance of trade. In addition, at a time when more than three million people are unemployed, at least 750,000 people are engaged in producing and selling alcohol.[22] A dramatic fall in consumption might mean a loss of Government income and lost jobs. Furthermore, the positive balance of payments resulting from alcohol sales may change quickly as we continue to drink more imported wine but lose exports as more countries in the world produce copies of our major alcoholic export, whisky. Alcohol abuse generates considerable costs, conservatively estimated at £1,700 million at 1983 prices.[26,27] This figure does not include the pain and suffering that are real but less easily measured costs of alcohol. In 1975 an estimate by the US government put the community cost at $43 billion in 1975;[28] in 1979, an economist estimated it to be in excess of $113 billion.[29] *Table 4* gives a list of the various social costs of alcohol abuse and *Table 5* shows the proportionate cost of its social consequences.

Physical Problems

Much (if not most) alcohol-related morbidity and mortality occurs in people who do not think of themselves, and may not be considered by their doctors, as either alcohol abusers or problem drinkers or dependent on alcohol.

Mortality

As many as 100,000 people a year in Britain may die prematurely because of tobacco smoking, but it is more difficult to estimate the number of premature deaths due to alcohol. Deaths due to cirrhosis and accidents, suicide, and other conditions associated with alcohol are grossly underestimated[30] – partly because doctors signing death certificates may be unwilling to invoke the stigma of alcohol abuse

Table 4 *Cost of alcohol abuse to the nation*

Cost to industry

1. Sickness absence.
2. Unexplained absence from the job and lateness to work.
3. Reduced efficiency and decision making at work.
4. Higher accident rates.
5. Impaired industrial relations.
6. Early retirement and premature death.
7. Higher labour turnover and retraining.

Cost to the NHS

1. Psychiatric care.
2. Non-psychiatric care.
3. GP care.

Social response costs

1. Expenditure by National alcohol bodies.
2. Research.

Cost of material damage

1. Road traffic accidents.
2. Home accidents, industrial accidents, and fire damage.

Cost of criminal activities

1. Police costs associated with traffic offences (excluding cost of accidents).
2. Other criminal offences.
3. Drink-related court cases.
4. Probation, judiciary and prison service.

Table 5 *Estimated social costs related to alcohol abuse in the United States, 1979*

category	$ m	%
lost production		
civilian	77,090	67
military	454	0.4
health care costs	20,465	18
motor vehicle crash costs	6,768	6
fire losses	647	0.6
violent crime	4,477	4
social response	3,467	3
Total	113,368	

(Adapted from Schifrin 1983.[29])

or, more importantly, because they may be unaware of the part played by alcohol. Recent changes in the Coroners' rules on death certification, excluding deaths due to chronic alcoholism from the need for an inquest, may encourage more accurate death certification.[31]

The official data for 1983 show that in England and Wales, 2184 people died of chronic liver disease and cirrhosis, in 887 of whom alcohol was given as a cause of death; 387 died in accidents where alcohol was mentioned (this excludes road accidents); 104 through 'non-dependent abuse of alcohol'; 99 of the alcohol dependency syndrome, and two from alcoholic psychosis.[32] About a third of deaths in road traffic accidents are associated with alcohol, i.e. about 1700 deaths a year (see p. 82).

Estimates of the total number of deaths from alcohol-related conditions have ranged from 5000 to 10,000 a year[8] and a recent estimate of the life years lost through alcohol in England and Wales in 1982 gives a low figure of 119,000 and a high figure of 192,000.[33] But even these may be underestimates, and the Royal College of General Practitioners has estimated that 40,000 deaths may be caused annually in Britain by alcohol.[22] Using the data from a study in Malmö, Sweden, of the death rate of 10,000 men whose drinking habits were known, it can be calculated that, in Britain among men aged 35–64, 25,000 deaths a year would be alcohol-related.[30,34] It has, moreover, been calculated that in Britain as many as 500 young people may die each year while drunk, representing 10 per cent of all deaths under 25.[35]

Alcohol misuse is also associated with sudden natural death. A study of 172 sudden, non-traumatic deaths in the United States showed that in sixteen individuals there was fatty change in the liver suggesting alcohol excess during life. The presence of a fatty liver was strongly associated with high blood alcohol levels at the time of death.[36]

Morbidity

Morbidity associated with alcohol excess is even more difficult to calculate. The Office of Health Economics has estimated that 8–15 million working days are lost each year in Britain because of alcohol-related illness.[8] The data from Malmö show that those men whose serum gamma glutamyl transpeptidase values (GGT, a biochemical marker of alcohol excess) were in the top tenth of the population, had about sixty sick days a year compared with twelve for those below the median.[37]

Hospitalization

In the Malmö study 963 of 4571 men born between 1926 and 1929 had spent 17,158 days in hospital within three years of screening, and 29 per cent of these days in hospital were for alcohol-related conditions.[30] In Britain and the United States a fifth of all acute male admissions to medical wards are associated with alcohol, 10–40 per cent of patients in general hospital beds are problem drinkers, and approximately one-third of patients attending casualty departments have a blood alcohol concentration above 80 mg/100 ml.[1-7,38] A recent study shows that more than a quarter (27 per cent) of 104 admissions to a general medical unit were attributed to alcohol but that only 10 of the 28 patients had classical alcohol-related conditions.[7]

A quarter of 949 cases of self-poisoning seen in sixty-two London casualty departments were associated with alcohol.[39] In Scotland, as many as two-thirds of cases of deliberate drug overdose may be associated with alcohol.[40]

Many elderly people, perhaps up to 60 per cent, who are admitted to hospital because of confusion, repeated falls at home, recurrent chest infections and heart failure, may have unrecognized alcohol problems.[41,42] Some of them are long-standing drinkers who have become old, others started drinking in old age, often after some major upheaval in their lives; elderly widowers are the most vulnerable group.

General Practice

Many people visit their general practitioners with alcohol-related problems.[43,44] It has been estimated that a general practitioner with 2000 patients would have 135 heavy drinkers, forty problem drinkers, and seven alcohol-dependent patients on his or her list.[44] But in one practice that had a disease register, only eighteen patients had been noted to be heavy drinkers.[45] This fits with other evidence that general practitioners, like hospital doctors, often fail to recognize the contribution made by alcohol to their patients' problems. This and other matters of alcohol-related problems in general practice are covered in the report of the Royal College of General Practitioners.[22]

Psychological Problems

The Royal College of Psychiatrists published its first report on alcohol problems in 1979,[13] and a second report has been published.[21] Because of this we will refer here only briefly to some of the mental health problems associated with excessive alcohol drinking. Many problems, such as depression, anxiety, personality disorders, hallucinations, and paranoid states are associated with alcohol in ways that are difficult to quantify at present.[46]

Psychiatrists have traditionally treated alcohol-related problems. In 1981 there were 17,955 alcohol-related admissions to mental hospitals in England and Wales – 12,026 for men and 5929 for women.[47] Just over 5000 were first admissions; just over 14,000 admissions in 1981 were for the alcohol dependency syndrome. An increasing proportion of patients are treated as outpatients: in Kent, the outpatient and day-patient rate is twelve times the inpatient rate.[48] In addition, many individuals do not come forward for treatment at all; those that do, may attend organizations like Alcoholics Anonymous or else receive treatment in non-psychiatric hospitals.

Suicide has been reported as being between twenty and almost sixty times more common among excessive drinkers than in the general population.[49-53] Between a quarter and a third of successful suicides occur in that group, and up to four-fifths of those who kill themselves have been drinking. A suicide attempt is more likely to be successful in an individual who has been drinking; those who are intoxicated are more likely to use more lethal methods.[53]

Family Problems

The families of problem drinkers possibly suffer as much as the individuals themselves. A third of problem drinkers list marital discord as one of their problems, and 40 per cent of cases brought before family courts in the United States involve alcohol abuse.[54] One-third of divorce petitions cite alcohol as a contributory factor.[54] Twenty-eight per cent of men in the Malmö study with GGT levels in the top tenth were divorced compared with only 3 per cent of those with concentrations in the lowest tenth.[30] As many as 80 per cent of cases of family violence in the United States involve alcohol.[54] Fifty-two husbands of 100 battered wives in Britain were 'frequently drunk' and in another twenty-two 'there were episodes of heavy drinking with drunkenness'.[55]

Conflict between parents is likely to affect children, and they may themselves be the direct recipients of violence associated with alcohol.[56-58] Neglect may be commoner than abuse because the dependent drinker is preoccupied with his or her drinking to the detriment of all else. Children may also be affected by poverty and debt caused by drinking (see Chapter 13).

Social Problems

The relation between alcohol and family and social problems is complicated; very rarely is a problem solely attributable to alcohol excess. This must be taken into account when considering the contribution of drinking to violence and crime.

In 1983 there were 109,724 convictions (101,120 men and 8604 women) and 2099 cautions for drunkenness in England and Wales.[59] In Scotland there were 11,328 convictions for drunkenness in 1981.

Occupation Problems

It has been estimated that most problem drinkers are still in full-time, gainful employment. These employees have an increased likelihood of accidents and a significantly higher level of absenteeism. A recent estimate has put the cost to industry of days lost through alcohol-related problems at £641 million a year (see Chapter 11).

Alcohol also affects judgement and decision making so that the obvious accidents on the shop floor may be paralleled by bad leadership and ineffective management through alcohol abuse in the board room or executive suite. These are largely invisible 'accidents', yet their effect may be more far-reaching than those confined to the shop floor.

Unemployment

The evidence on whether unemployed people drink more or less alcohol is confusing. Some studies suggest that they drink more [60,61] and some that they drink less,[62] while others have found no relation between unemployment and alcohol consumption.[63] These contradictory results may be explained by methodological weaknesses, but recent work also shows that while most of the unemployed drink less because of relative poverty, a minority drink much more.[64,65] An explanation may be found in the definition of unemployed: the

Scottish OPCS study[66] showed a 28 per cent drop in unemployed men's consumption, but a rise in retired men's consumption of 56 per cent. Recent work has also suggested that the style of drinking rather than the amount may be affected by unemployment. Crawford et al.[65] looked at the drinking habits of 87 unemployed men among 1503 economically active men and found that the unemployed drank the same amount as the employed in the week of the survey but drank faster, were more likely to have had a heavy drinking day and a binge, and suffered more consequences from their drinking.

None of this research has been able to determine whether it is the unemployment itself that causes the changes in alcohol consumption. It may be that the change comes before – and even contributes to – unemployment, or it may be that some other factor is related to both unemployment and drinking habits.

Homelessness

Out of 158 men who came to the Bureau for Homeless Men in Stockholm, 150 had records of alcohol problems, 145 exhibited signs of alcohol dependence, and 106 had at least seven convictions for drunkenness.[79] Among 79 men living in an Edinburgh lodging house, 18 per cent were definitely or probably abusing alcohol, as were 34 per cent of 44 men in similar circumstances who were admitted to hospital. There may be more than 100,000 homeless people (mostly men) in Britain,[80] many with severe alcohol problems as part of their social incapacity.

Driving Offences

In 1982, there were 63,832 convictions for drinking and driving offences in England and Wales (61,099 men and 2733 women),[67] and 11,244 in Scotland in 1981.[69] Only 12 per cent of those convicted in England and Wales had blood alcohol concentrations between 81 and 100 mg/100 ml, while 56 per cent had concentrations above 150 mg/100 ml.[68] Thus, many people who drive with blood concentrations of alcohol only just over the legal limit of 80 mg/100 ml are probably not convicted, which fits with a Home Office study that suggests that only one in 250 episodes of drunken driving results in a conviction.[69] This, too, is likely to be a conservative estimate, because many people are not enthusiastic about telling the Home Office how often they have driven while over the legal limit.

Other Offences

Alcohol misuse is also strongly associated with crime against persons and property. In 18 of 28 studies which investigated homicide, more than half of the offenders had been drinking at the time they committed the offence.[70] In the West of Scotland more than half of 400 people found guilty of homicide were intoxicated when they committed the murder and more than half their victims were also intoxicated.[71] A similar study in Helsinki found that almost four-fifths of the murderers and their victims were intoxicated;[72] of seventy-seven convicted rapists in the United States half were drinking when they committed the offence and more than a third were classed as alcohol abusers.[73]

In three of six studies on burglary more than half the offenders had been drinking immediately before they committed the offence.[74] Two-thirds of a group of 121 British offenders serving sentences for burglary had drunk alcohol before at least one burglary, and about a third said that their offences were usually committed under the influence of alcohol.[74]

Prisoners have a high incidence of alcohol-related problems. Of 1420 admissions to New York correctional facilities in 1975, 18 per cent of the men and 14 per cent of the women had a history of alcohol abuse.[77] Forty-one per cent of 638 women admitted to Holloway prison in 1967 for failing to pay a fine were alcohol abusers.[78]

Football supporters may be one group of people in whom alcohol abuse and violence are associated. An investigation carried out by the Birmingham Research Group in the 1960s in response to a request by the then Minister of Sport[75,76] concluded that alcohol contributed considerably to the problem in Scotland and the North of England but not so much in the South: 20 of 74 police authorities thought that alcohol was important, 11 in Scotland, but only one in the South of England. One Scottish police officer told the group that of 110 men arrested at one match 93 had been drinking and 17 had not. But it was also stated that alcohol was not important as a contributory factor in those under eighteen.

References

1. Jarman, C.M.B. and Kellett, J.M. (1979) Alcoholism in the General Hospital. *British Medical Journal* ii: 469–71.

2. Quinn, M. and Johnstone, R. (1976) Alcohol Problems in Acute Male Medical Admissions. *Health Bulletin* 34: 253.
3. McCusker, J., Cherubin, C.E., and Zimberg, S. (1979) Prevalence of Alcoholism in a General Municipal Hospital Population. *New York State Journal of Medicine* 3: 751–54.
4. Moore, R.A. (1971) Prevalence of Alcoholism in a Community General Hospital. *American Journal of Psychiatry* 128: 638–39.
5. Jaswrilla, A.G., Adams, P.H., and Hore, B.D. (1979) Alcohol and Acute General Medical Admissions. *Health Trends* 11: 95–7.
6. Barrison, I.G., Viola, L., Mumford, J., Murray, R.M., Gordon, M., and Murray-Lyon, I.M. (1982) Detecting Excessive Drinking Among Admissions to a General Hospital. *Health Trends* 14: 80–3.
7. Lockhart, S.P., Carter, Y.H., Straffen, A.M., Pang, K.K., McLoughlin, J., and Baron, J.H. (1986) Detecting Alcohol Consumption as a Cause of Emergency General Medical Admissions. *Journal of the Royal Society of Medicine* 79: 558.
8. Taylor, D. (1981) *Alcohol: Reducing the Harm.* London: Office of Health Economics.
9. Lloyd, G., Chick, J., Crombie, E., and Anderson, S. (1986) Problem Drinkers in Medical Wards: Consumption Patterns and Disabilities in Newly Identified Male Cases. *British Journal of Addiction* (December).
10. Barrison, I.G., Viola, L., and Murray-Lyon, I.M. (1980) Do Housemen Take an Adequate Drinking History? *British Medical Journal* 281: 1040.
11. Flaherty, J.A. and Flaherty, E.G. (1983) Medical Students' Performance in Reporting Alcohol-Related Problems. *Journal of the Study of Alcohol* 44: 1083–087.
12. Anonymous (1984) Drink. *Which?* October: 445–49.
13. Special Committee of the Royal College of Psychiatrists (1979) *Alcohol and Alcoholism.* London: Tavistock Publications.
14. World Health Organisation Expert Committee (1979) *Problems Related to Alcohol Consumption.* Geneva: WHO.
15. House of Commons Expenditure Committee (1977) *Report on Preventive Medicine.* London: HMSO.
16. Brunn, K. (1982) *Alcohol Policies in the United Kingdom.* Stockholm: Sociologiska Institution.
17. Department of Health and Social Security Advisory Committee of Alcoholism (1978) *Report on Prevention.* London: HMSO.
18. Department of Health and Social Security (1981) *Prevention and Health; Drinking Sensibly.* London: HMSO.
19. Robertson, I., Hodgson, R., Orford, J., and McKechnie, R. (1984) *Psychology and Problem Drinking.* Report of a working party convened by the British Psychological Society Division of Clinical Psychology. Leicester: BPS.
20. Scottish Health Education Co-ordinating Committee (1985) *Health Education in the Prevention of Alcohol-Related Problems.* Edinburgh: Scottish Home and Health Department.
21. Special Committee of the Royal College of Psychiatrists (1986) *Alcohol – Our Favourite Drug.* London: Tavistock Publications.

22. Royal College of General Practitioners (1986) *Alcohol – A Balanced View*. London: Royal College of General Practitioners.
23. Valliant, G.E. (1980) The Doctor's Dilemma. In G. Edwards and M. Grant (eds) *Alcohol Treatment in Transition*. London: Croom Helm.
24. Saunders, W.M. (1984) Alcohol Use in Britain: How Much is Too Much? *Health Education Journal* 43: 66–70.
25. Hayhoe, B. (1985) Parliamentary written answer. House of Commons Official Report (Hansard), 12 November 67: col. 88.
26. Maynard, A. (1984) The Social Costs of Alcohol Use. In *Alcohol: Preventing the Harm*. London: Institute of Alcohol Studies.
27. McDonnell, R. and Maynard, A. (1985) The Costs of Alcohol Misuse. *British Journal of Addiction* 80: 27–35.
28. Berry, R.E., Boland, J.P., Smart, C.N. and Knak, J.R. (1977) *The Economic Costs of Alcohol Abuse – 1975*. Washington: National Institute of Alcohol Abuse and Alcoholism.
29. Schifrin, L.G. (1983) Social Costs of Alcohol Abuse in the United States: an Updating. In M. Grant, M. Plant, and A. Williams (eds) *Economics and Alcohol*. London: Croom Helm.
30. Kristenson, H. and Hood, B. (1984) The Impact of Alcohol on Health in the General Population: a Review with Particular Reference to Experience in Malmö. *British Journal of Addiction* 79: 139–45.
31. Maxwell, J.D. and Knapman, P. (1985) Effect of Coroners' Rules on Death Certification for Alcoholic Liver Disease. *British Medical Journal* 291: 708.
32. Short, R. (1985) Parliamentary written answer. House of Commons Official Report (Hansard) 17 January 71: col. 216–18.
33. McDonnell, R. and Maynard, A. (1985) Estimation of Life Years Lost From Alcohol Related Premature Deaths. *Alcohol and Alcoholism* 20: 435–43.
34. Peterson, B., Krantz, P., Kristenson, H., Trell, E., and Sternby, N.H. (1982) Alcohol Related Death: a Major Contributor to Mortality in Urban Middle-Aged Men. *Lancet* 11: 1088–090.
35. Sabey, B. and Coding, P. (1975) Alcohol and Road Accidents in Great Britain. In S. Israelstam and S. Lamber (eds) *Alcohol, Drugs and Road Safety*. Toronto: Addiction Research Foundation.
36. May, S.J., Kuller, L.H., and Perper, J.A. (1980) The Relationship of Alcohol to Sudden Natural Death: an Epidemiological Analysis. *Journal of the Study of Alcohol* 41: 693–701.
37. Kristenson, H., Ohrn, J., Trell, E., and Hood, B. (1980) Serum Gamma Glutamyltransferase at Screening and Retrospective Sick Days. *Lancet* 1: 1141.
38. Holt, S., Stewart, I.C., Dixon, J.M.J., Elton, R.A., Taylor, T.V., and Little, K. (1980) Alcohol and the Emergency Service Patient. *British Medical Journal* 281: 638–40.
39. Ghodse, A.H. (1980) Deliberate Self-Poisoning: a Study in London Casualty Departments. *British Medical Journal* i: 805–08.
40. Platt, S. (1984) Cited in W. M. Saunders (ed.) Alcohol Use in Britain: How Much is Too Much? *Health Education Journal* 43: 66–70.

41. Wattis, J.P. (1981) Alcohol Problems in the Elderly. *Journal of the American Geriatrics Society* 29: 131–34.
42. Glatt, M.M., Rosin, A.J., and Jauhar, P. (1978) Alcoholic Problems in the Elderly. *Age and Ageing* 7: Suppl. 64.
43. Wilkins, R.H. (1974) *The Hidden Alcoholic in General Practice.* London: Elek Science.
44. Anderson, P. (1983) Alcohol. In S. Lock (ed.) *Practising Prevention.* London: British Medical Association.
45. Wallace, P. and Haines, A. (1985) The Use of a Questionnaire in General Practice to Increase the Recognition of Patients with Excessive Alcohol Consumption. *British Medical Journal* 29: 1949–952.
46. Thorley, A. (1982) The Effects of Alcohol. In M. A. Plant (ed.) *Drinking and Problem Drinking.* London: Junction Books.
47. Department of Health and Social Security (1984) *Statistical Note: Alcohol Misuse: Results from the Mental Health Enquiry.* London: DHSS.
48. Latcham, R.W., Kreitman, N., Plant, M.A., and Crawford, A. (1984) Regional Variations in British Alcohol Morbidity Rates: a Myth Uncovered? I. Clinical Surveys. *British Medical Journal* 289: 1341–343.
49. Maull, K.I. (1982) Alcohol Abuse: Its Implications in Trauma Care. *Southern Medical Journal* 75: 794–98.
50. Medhus, A. (1975) Mortality Among Female Alcoholics. *Scandinavian Journal of Social Medicine* 3: 11–15.
51. Woodruff, R.A., Goodwin, D., and Guze, S. (1974) *Psychiatric Diagnosis.* New York: Oxford University Press.
52. O'Brien, R. and Chafetz, M. (1982) *The Encyclopedia of Alcoholism.* London: Library Association.
53. Beck, A.T., Wissman, A., and Kovacs, M. (1976) Alcoholism, Hopelessness, and Suicidal Behaviour. *Journal of the Study of Alcohol* 37: 66–77.
54. Jacob, T. and Seilhamer, R.A. (1982) The Impact on Spouses and How They Cope. In J. Orford and J. Harwin (eds) *Alcohol and the Family.* London: Croom Helm.
55. Gayford, J.J. (1975) Wife Battering: a Preliminary Survey of 100 Cases. *British Medical Journal* i: 194–97.
56. Wilson, C. (1982) The Impact on Children. In J. Orford and J. Harwin (eds) *Alcohol and the Family.* London: Croom Helm.
57. Mayer, J. and Black, R. (1977) The Relationship Between Alcoholism and Child Abuse and Neglect. In F. A. Seixas (ed.) *Currents in Alcoholism, Vol. 2. Psychiatric, Social and Epidemiological Studies.* New York: Grune and Stratton.
58. Smith, S.M., Hanson, R., and Noble, S. (1973) Parents of Battered Babies: a Controlled Study. *British Medical Journal* iv: 388–91.
59. Home Office (1984) *Offences of Drunkenness, England and Wales 1983.* London: HMSO.
60. Office of Population Censuses and Surveys. (1984) *General Household Survey 1982.* London: HMSO.
61. Cobb, S. and Kasl, S.V. (1977) *Termination: the Consequence of Job Loss.*

Washington, DC: National Institute for Occupational Safety and Health.
62. Plant, M.A. (1979) *Drinking Careers: Occupations, Drinking Habits, and Drinking Problems*. London: Tavistock Publications.
63. Cook, D.G., Cummins, R.O., Bartley, M.J., and Shaper, A.G. (1982) Health of Unemployed Middle-Aged Men in Great Britain. *Lancet* i: 1290–294.
64. Yates, F., Hebblethwaithe, F., and Thorley, A. (1984) *Drinking in Two North East Towns: a Survey of the Natural Setting for Prevention*. Newcastle upon Tyne: Centre for Alcohol and Drug Studies.
65. Crawford, M.A., Plant, M.A., Kreitman, N., and Latcham, R.W. (in preparation) Unemployment and Drinking Behaviour: Some Data from a General Population Survey of Alcohol Use.
66. Goddard, E. (1985) *Drinking and Attitudes to Licensing in Scotland*. London: HMSO.
67. Home Office. (1983) *Offences Relating to Motor Vehicles, England and Wales*. London: HMSO.
68. Brewers' Society (1983) *United Kingdom Statistical Handbook*. London: Brewers' Society.
69. Riley, D. (1984) *Drivers' Beliefs about Alcohol and the Law*. Home Office Research Bulletin, No. 17. London: Home Office.
70. Greenberg, S.W. (1982) Alcohol and Crime: a Methodological Critique of the Literature. In J. J. Collins (ed.) *Drinking and Crime: Perspectives on the Relationships between Alcohol Consumption and Criminal Behaviour*. London: Tavistock Publications.
71. Gillies, H. (1976) Homicide in the West of Scotland. *British Medical Journal* 128: 105–27.
72. Hagnell, O., Nyman, E., and Tunvirg, K. (1973) Dangerous Alcoholics. *Scandinavian Journal of Social Medicine* 3: 125–31.
73. Rada, R.T. (1975) Alcoholism and Forcible Rape. *American Journal of Psychiatry* 132: 444–46.
74. Bennett, T. and Wright, R. (1984) The Relationship Between Alcohol Use and Burglary. *British Journal of Addiction* 79: 431–37.
75. Birmingham Research Group (1968) *A Preliminary Report on Soccer Hooliganism*. Bristol: Wrights.
76. Parliamentary All Party Penal Affairs Group (1984) *The Prevention of Crime Among Young People*. London: PAPAG.
77. Novick, L.F., Penna, R.D., Schwartz, M.S., Remmlinger, E., and Loewenstein, R. (1977) Health Status of the New York Prison Population. *Medical Care* 15: 205–16.
78. Gibben, T.C.N. (1971) Female Offenders. *British Journal of Hospital Medicine* 6: 279–90.
79. Borg, S. (1978) Homeless Men. A Clinical and Social Study with Special Reference to Alcohol Abuse. *Acta Psychologica Scandinavica* Supplementum 276.
80. Priest, R.G. (1976) The Homeless Person and the Psychiatric Services: an Edinburgh Survey. *British Journal of Psychiatry* 128: 128–36.

2

LEVELS OF ALCOHOL CONSUMPTION IN BRITAIN

Summary

Consumption of beer, wines, and spirits has risen sharply in the UK during the past thirty years. People's drinking habits are a product of interacting personal and environmental influences. These include age, sex, occupation, income, marital status, as well as the cost and availability of alcoholic drinks. Mortality from cirrhosis of the liver is one of the most useful indicators of trends in alcohol-related disease and has risen and fallen in parallel with alcohol consumption. Incidence and mortality from a range of other diseases also varies with the per capita consumption levels of populations. The relationship between levels of individual consumption and the development of disease is more difficult to assess.

Patterns of Drinking

Britain is traditionally a beer drinking country. During 1983 the average annual consumption of alcoholic drinks per person aged fifteen years and over was 138 litres (243 pints) of beer, 12 litres of wine, 7 litres (1.5 gallons) of cider, and 5 litres of spirits.[1] This did not take account of home brewed beverages, which included 204 million litres (360 million pints) of beer and 240,000 litres (9 million pints) of wine made from 'kits'. Total consumption of pure alcohol was almost 9 litres per year and provided 6 per cent of average energy intake derived from food.[2]

During the first half of this century there was a fall in beer consumption, initiated at the time of the First World War[3] (*Figure 2*). Consumption rose sharply in the Second World War, fell during the post-war period and rose again from 1960 onwards. During the last decade it was at its highest level for sixty years, reaching five pints per week per person aged fifteen or over in 1978–79.

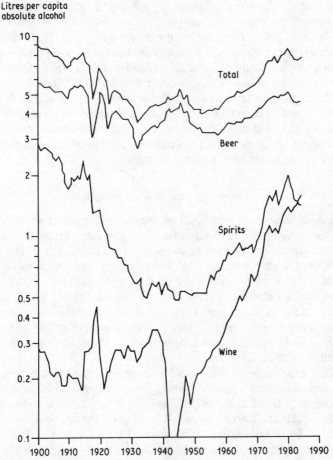

Litres per capita
absolute alcohol

Figure 2 Changes in alcohol consumption per person from 1900 to 1986.

In contrast, spirits drinking declined steadily throughout the first half of the century to reach low levels during the Second World War. From around 1950 consumption rose again, and was accompanied by an increase in wine drinking. In the past twenty years spirits consumption has more than doubled and wine consumption has quadrupled. These increases, occurring in addition to, rather than in replacement of, beer, follow a pattern observed in many other countries. When alcohol intake increases, an overlay of 'international' drinking is superimposed on traditional habits.[4]

In 1983 regional expenditure on alcoholic drinks was highest in

Wales and Northern England (£7.08 and £7.19 respectively per
household per week) and least in East Anglia and Northern Ireland
(£4.70 and £3.63). The greatest differences were in the expenditure on
beer, £5.21 per household per week in the northern region compared
with £1.58 in Northern Ireland; spirits and wines ranged from £2.58
in Greater London to £1.40 in Northern Ireland.[5] One-third of the
men in Northern Ireland and half the women are teetotal, compared
with figures of 6 and 11 per cent for men and women elsewhere in
the United Kingdom.[6] These regional differences cannot be
accounted for by differences in income, total consumer expenditure,
age, sex, or other demographic variables.

Determinants of Consumption

Drinking habits are a product of interacting personal and environmental influences. In England and Wales men drink on average
more than twice as much as women – 19.6 units (157 g) per week
compared with 7 units (56 g)[6] – and young men drink more than
older men – 26.6 units (213 g) per week at ages 20–27 years
compared with 20 units (160 g) in middle age (28–57 years) and 14
units (112 g) at older ages. Likewise young women drink more than
older women – 9.7 units (78 g) per week at ages 20–27 compared
with 5 units (40 g) at older ages. Married people drink less than
single men and women.

The effects of income and occupation on consumption are
interrelated. For example, among married men in non-manual
occupations those in the middle income group drink less than those
with higher and lower incomes.[6] In manual occupations, however,
the middle income group drink more.

Consumption may be analysed in terms of the proportions of
people with intakes above a given level.[6,7] Patterns for age, sex, and
marital status are similar to those for average consumption, but
differences between occupational groups are revealed. For example,
there is a higher percentage of men drinking more than 50 units
(400 g) a week in manual than non-manual occupations. The highest
percentage of heavier drinkers reported in the 1982 General
Household Survey was among unemployed men aged 18–44 years.[7]
However, a recent survey in Scotland showed no marked association
between employment status and alcohol consumption, except that,
not unexpectedly, habitually heavy drinkers appeared to be at
greater risk of losing their jobs at a time of rising unemployment.[8]

Consumption levels in populations, as opposed to individuals, are influenced by cost, availability, and possibly advertising. There are many instances of consumption rising when the cost of alcohol, relative to the standard of living, falls.[9-11] In Britain the rise in consumption during the past thirty years has been associated with increasing prosperity. In March 1981 an increase in excise duty caused the price of alcohol to rise faster than incomes. A sample of regular drinkers in Scotland was interviewed on two occasions, before and after the increase. Their alcohol consumption fell by 18 per cent. The main determinant was the price increase.[8] Consumption rises in the face of price increases if the level of disposable income rises more rapidly, as in Ireland during 1960–74.[12]

Governments in Britain and elsewhere have manipulated national consumption levels by legislating on the importation of alcoholic beverages, duties and excise, licensing hours and numbers of licensed premises, legal age of drinking, and even the growth of crops used for fermentation. Licensing hours influence the pattern of drinking but do not necessarily change consumption levels. Average consumption in Scotland is similar to that in England and Wales. However, in the past, shorter licensing hours in Scotland resulted in more rapid drinking.[6] Forty per cent of male Scottish drinkers reported having 'heavy drinking days' (more than 8 units) compared with 27 per cent of male drinkers in England and Wales.

Advertising may influence consumption levels, but its role is unclear.[9] It may affect the choice of drink and the pattern of drinking more than total consumption.

The relationship between environmental and personal influences on consumption levels has been assessed primarily by the use of sample surveys, all of which estimate average alcohol consumption to be only 40–60 per cent of that calculated by Customs and Excise. This shortfall arises for a number of reasons, including exclusion of heavy drinkers from sampling frames (for example if they have no fixed abode), poor compliance of heavy drinkers in surveys, poor recall of consumption (especially for drinks at home when standard measures are not used), and deliberate under-reporting.

New techniques, such as 'interviews' with microcomputers with interactive programmes, may help to overcome these problems.

Levels of Consumption and Disease in Populations

Mortality from alcoholism and cirrhosis of the liver (*Figure 3*), derived from deaths in which these are certified as the underlying cause,[3] is the most widely used indicator of the incidence of alcohol-

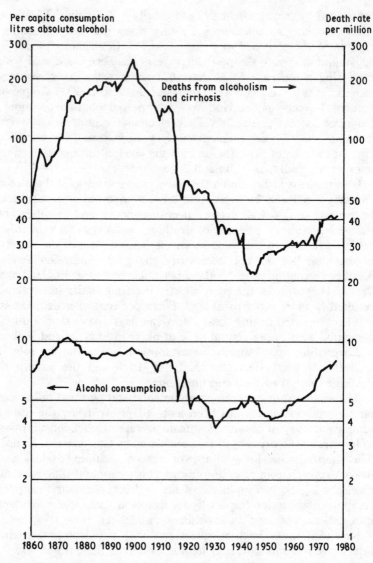

Figure 3 Trends in alcohol consumption and deaths attributed to alcohol.

related disease in populations. Although interpretation is complicated by several factors such as the known under-recording of alcoholism on death certificates (see p. 8), the high cirrhosis rates in occupations in which people are known to drink heavily, for example publicans, support the view that it is a valid indicator. Changes in mortality rates in England and Wales from 1860 to 1978 paralleled those in alcohol consumption. In particular, the rise in consumption from 1950 was associated with a progressive rise in cirrhosis mortality. Rates for men were consistently higher than for women. The proportion of deaths from cirrhosis certified as due to alcoholic cirrhosis rose steeply after 1950.[13] Additional evidence that the rise in cirrhosis was due mainly to alcohol-related disease rather than other causes comes from one local survey. During 1959–76 the incidence of alcoholic cirrhosis in the West Midlands increased by around three times, whereas the incidence of other forms of cirrhosis was constant.[14]

Alcohol also contributes to a wide range of other medical problems, but data which allow comparison of trends in its consumption and in the alcohol component of these disorders are sparse. The rise in UK consumption during 1970–79 was accompanied by a rise in mortality from oesophageal and pancreatic cancer. In Finland, increasing consumption from 1950–75 was associated with increasing alcohol-related traffic accidents, crimes of assault, and deaths from alcohol poisoning, as well as increasing cirrhosis mortality.[15] In Copenhagen, increasing consumption during the 1970s was accompanied by a rise in the incidence of chronic pancreatitis.[16]

Geographical comparisons give additional evidence of a relationship between individual consumption levels and disease rates. Differences in alcohol consumption between eighteen European countries during the 1970s correlate with variations in mortality from cirrhosis of the liver (*Figure 4*).[3]

Differences in consumption within Europe also parallel mortality rates from cancer of the oesophagus.[17] Within England and Wales there are correlations at regional level between hospital admission rates for alcoholism, alcohol-related crime rates, and mortality from alcohol-related diseases, such as alcoholic psychosis, persistent alcohol abuse, alcoholic poisoning, cirrhosis, and suicide.[18] Comparisons between twenty-four British towns have shown that the proportion of heavy drinkers, that is people who drink more than six units either daily or on each day at the weekend, is positively correlated with mortality from coronary heart disease.[19]

Available data therefore point to positive associations between the per capita consumption levels of populations and mortality and incidence rates for a range of alcohol-related diseases. The strength

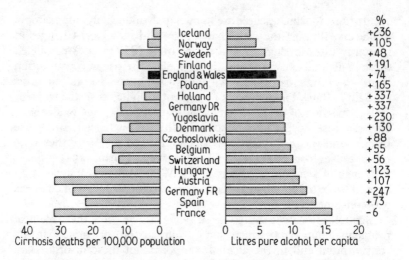

Figure 4 Changes in alcohol consumption, 1950–52 to mid–1970s.

of these relationships must be affected by the drinking patterns and distributions of consumption within the populations.

Consumption and Ill-Health in Individuals

What is the relationship between levels of individual consumption and the development of disease? Much of our knowledge of the adverse effects of alcohol comes from studies on 'alcoholics'. Interpretation of these studies is, however, difficult. There are problems with definitions as we have indicated, and excessive drinkers are exposed not only to the effects of high alcohol intake but also to other adverse influences, such as dietary deficiencies and cigarette smoking. Simple observation shows that alcohol intake below intoxicating levels may lead to traffic accidents, accidents at work, other forms of trauma, gastritis, and impotence. The problems of studying possible deleterious effects of moderate alcohol intake therefore centre on the chronic, rather than the acute effects.

Measurement of patterns and amounts of drinking depends on the memory and responses of individuals at interview. Therefore the accuracy of data is often in question. This is a major obstacle to establishing levels of drinking which do not impair physical health. The need for recommendations on levels of consumption rather than abstinence, arises from the social value of alcohol, real or perceived, but has been reinforced by findings which suggest that abstainers do not necessarily enjoy better health than moderate drinkers (see pp. 8 and 59). However, abstainers are an unusual group – only 6 per cent of men in England and Wales describe themselves as non-drinkers. They include lifetime abstainers and those who have given up drinking for various reasons, which may include incipient illness. It is possible that non-drinkers differ from moderate drinkers in ways other than the frequency of major risk factors which put them at higher risk of heart disease, for example personality type or diet. At present there is insufficient evidence to resolve this and it remains possible that moderate drinking is protective.

References

1. Central Statistical Office (1984) *Monthly Digest of Statistics: December 1984*. London: HMSO.
2. Ministry of Agriculture, Fisheries and Food (1984) *Household Food Consumption and Expenditure: 1982*. London: HMSO.
3. Taylor, D. (1981) *Alcohol: Reducing the Harm*. London: Office of Health Economics.
4. World Health Organisation (1980) *Problems Related to Alcohol Consumption*. Technical Report Series No. 650. Geneva: WHO.
5. Department of Employment (1984) *Family Expenditure Survey: 1982*. London: HMSO.
6. Wilson, P. (1980) Drinking Habits in the United Kingdom. *Population Trends* 22: 14–18.
7. Office of Population Censuses and Surveys (1984) *General Household Survey: 1982*. London: HMSO.
8. Kendell, R.E., de Roumanie, M. and Ritson, E.B. (1983) Effect of Economic Changes on Scottish Drinking Habits 1978–82. *British Journal of Addiction* 78: 305–79.
9. Smith, R. (1981) Alcohol and Alcoholism: the Relation Between Consumption and Damage. *British Medical Journal* 282: 895–98.
10. Spring, J.A. and Buss, D.H. (1977) Three Centuries of Alcohol in the British Diet. *Nature* 270: 567–72.
11. Kendell, R.E. (1984) The Beneficial Consequence of the United Kingdom's Declining Per Capita Consumption of Alcohol in 1979–82. *Alcohol and Alcoholism* 19: 271–76.
12. Walsh, B.M. (1980) *Drinking in Ireland*. Dublin: Dublin Economic and Social Research Institute.
13. Donnan, S. and Haskey, J. (1977) Alcoholism and Cirrhosis of the Liver. *Population Trends* 7: 18–24.
14. Saunders, J.B., Walters, J.R.F., Davies, P., and Paton, A. (1981) A 20 Year Prospective Study of Cirrhosis. *British Medical Journal* 282: 263–66.
15. Osterberg, E. (1979) *Recorded Consumption of Alcohol in Finland, 1950–75*. Helsinki: Social Research Institute of Alcohol Studies.

16. Andersen, B.N., Pedersen, N.T., Scheek, J., and Worning, H. (1982) Incidence of Alcoholic Chronic Pancreatitis in Copenhagen. *Scandinavian Journal of Gastroenterology* 17: 247–52.
17. Audigier, J.C., Tuyns, A.J., and Lambert, R. (1975) Epidemiology of Oesophageal Cancer in France. Increasing Mortality and Persistent Correlation with Alcoholism. *Digestion* 13: 209–19.
18. Kilich, S. and Plant, M. (1981) Regional Variations in the Levels of Alcohol-Related Problems in Britain. *British Journal of Addiction* 76: 47–62.
19. Shaper, A.G., Pocock, S.J., Walker, M., Cohen, N.M., Wale, C.J., and Thomson, A.G. (1981) British Regional Heart Study: Cardiovascular Risk Factors in Middle-aged Men in 24 Towns. *British Medical Journal* 283: 179–86.

3

THE NERVOUS SYSTEM

Summary

The deleterious effects of alcohol abuse on the nervous system can be subdivided into three categories:

1. Acute intoxication;
2. The consequences of withdrawal after habituation, the commonest of which are alcoholic tremor, seizures and delirium tremens;
3. Conditions related to prolonged abuse.

Some of these, such as Wernicke's encephalopathy, Korsakoff's syndrome and alcoholic peripheral nerve damage are predominantly related to secondary vitamin deficiency; others are the result of alcohol-induced disease of the brain and its blood vessels or of the liver. Together these effects comprise frequent and often serious causes of neurological and psychiatric disease.

Alcohol is consumed for its effect on the nervous system. It is not surprising, therefore, that neurological disturbances are prominent among the adverse effects of excessive intake.

Acute Intoxication

The behavioural consequences of alcoholic intoxication are summarized in *Table 6*. Alcohol depresses nerve cell activity, the initial effects probably being related to disturbances of brainstem and cerebellar function, the cerebral cortex being affected later. During the stage of inebriation, the personality of the individual and the environment at

Table 6 *Effects and blood alcohol level of specific quantities of alcohol intake*

number of drinks	blood alcohol level (mg/100ml)	effects
1 pint of beer or 2 glasses of wine or a double whisky	30	increasing likelihood of having an accident
1.5 pints beer or 3 whiskies or half a (75 cl) bottle of wine	50	increasing cheerfulness, impaired judgement and loosening of inhibitions
2.5 pints of beer or 5 whiskies or 5 glasses of wine	80	loss of driving licence if caught
5 pints of beer or 10 whiskies or 1 litre of wine	150	loss of self-control; exuberance; quarrelsomeness; slurred speech
6 pints of beer or half a bottle of spirits or 2 (75 cl) bottles of wine	200	stagger; double vision; loss of memory
0.75 bottle of spirits	400	oblivion; sleepiness; coma
1 bottle of spirits	500	death possible
	600	death certain

(Adapted from *Helping You to Better Health*, Health Education Council, London: HEC)

the time play an important part. In congenial company the drinker often feels excited and elated, becomes more loquacious, and loses some of the normal social inhibitions. Solitary drinking may lead to feelings of depression and social isolation. With advancing intoxication come slurring of speech, unsteadiness and drowsiness, accompanied by autonomic effects such as flushing of the skin, dilatation of the pupils, and a fast heart rate. At this stage, reasoning and memory become increasingly impaired, perception is reduced, and the individual becomes readily distractable. Reduced motor and intellectual performance conflicts with feelings of enhanced ability. The individual loses emotional restraint and becomes excessively and sometimes inappropriately jocular, aggressive and occasionally paranoid, or full of self-pity. More severe intoxication leads to increasing drowsiness and then coma, with depressed tendon reflexes, low blood pressure, and low body temperature. Respiration becomes slow and stertorous. The pupils may be dilated or constricted. Death may result from respiratory depression or, at an earlier stage of intoxication, from inhalation of vomit.

Blood alcohol levels necessary to produce intoxication depend upon the rate of intake, the degree of tolerance acquired by previous regular consumption of alcohol and the simultaneous effects of other drugs. A rapid rise in the blood alcohol level produces a greater degree of intoxication than a gradual rise to the same level and substantial tolerance develops in regular drinkers.[1] In non-habituated subjects, a level of 150–250 mg/100ml generally gives rise to obvious intoxication and even concentrations of 31–65 mg/100ml lead to definite impairment of cognitive function, motor coordination, and sensory perception. On the other hand, in regular drinkers, levels of more than 500 mg/100 ml may be present without signs of inebriation. The speed with which tolerance is established is evidenced by the fact that sobriety returns at blood alcohol levels that caused intoxication during prior acute intake.[2] Experimentally, tolerance by the nervous system has been shown to occur within as short a period as thirty minutes.[3]

'Black-Outs'

All subjects will necessarily lose memory for periods during which consciousness has been impaired. Individuals occasionally develop alcoholic 'black-outs' consisting of loss of memory for several hours, sometimes for several days, but during these episodes they may appear to behave relatively normally.

Sometimes there is associated fugue-like behaviour, the individual characteristically travelling long distances and regaining normality with no knowledge as to how he or she has arrived elsewhere.[4] Behaviour appears relatively normal and subjectively the attacks have an abrupt onset and termination. The mechanism of these attacks is obscure; some may represent secondary psychiatric reactions, but most do not.

Alcohol-Withdrawal Effects

Complete or partial abstinence after prolonged and regular, heavy intake creates a range of phenomena, including tremor, hallucinations, withdrawal seizures and delirium tremens. The likelihood of their occurrence and severity is directly related to the duration and

magnitude of the preceding intake. In a consecutive series of 266
patients admitted to the Boston City Hospital with neurological
complications of alcoholism, acute tremor occurred in 34 per cent,
withdrawal seizures in 12 per cent, tremor and hallucinations in 11
per cent, delirium tremens in 5 per cent, and auditory hallucinations
in 2 per cent.[5]

Tremor

Trembling is the most consistent manifestation of withdrawal and
may be observed after a drinking bout lasting a few days. In mild
form it is often present in chronic alcohol abusers on waking in the
morning before the first drink of the day. In more severe instances,
increasing tremor appears 12–24 hours after the last drink and is
most obtrusive in the upper limbs. It is accompanied by feelings of
restlessness and agitation and insomnia and the subject is easily
startled. The tremor is promptly relieved by further alcohol intake
but would otherwise subside spontaneously within hours or days,
depending upon its severity.

Hallucinations

Auditory hallucinations ('hearing voices') develop as a rare manifestation within a few days of alcohol withdrawal. Initially there may
be nondescript sounds such as buzzing or ringing in the ears, which
then evolve into verbal form, often with an unpleasant or accusatory
content, occurring on a background of full consciousness. They
usually appear when intake is being curtailed but in rare instances
they appear while the individual is still drinking. In the majority of
instances the sounds subside within hours or days; sometimes they
continue for several months and occasionally are persistent. When
persistent, the precipitation of latent schizophrenia seems likely.

Delirium Tremens

Although milder manifestations may occur, the complete syndrome
represents a serious disorder that develops 2–5 days after alcohol
withdrawal. The onset is often abrupt, frequently at night, but may
be preceded by increasing restlessness and feelings of apprehension,
nightmares, and mental disorientation. Once the condition is
established, the subject trembles and is agitated, with fear increasing

to panic as he or she wakes in terror from vivid nightmares. The individual becomes increasingly restless, confused, and disorientated and begins to experience hallucinations. These are predominantly visual and characteristically of animal life. Persecutory auditory hallucinations may occur. Illusory phenomena may also be observed so that marks on the bed linen or walls, for example, may be interpreted as crawling insects. Mostly the hallucinations and illusions generate fear, sometimes amusement. These behavioural changes are associated with autonomic manifestations, including sweating, fast pulse, skin flushing or pallor, and fever.

Delirium tremens usually subsides in 2–3 days but has a significant morbidity and mortality due to injuries sustained during the period of confusion, and from dehydration and circulatory collapse, hypothermia, and intercurrent pneumonia.

Withdrawal Seizures

Isolated or repeated generalized epileptic seizures, sometimes status epilepticus, are usually encountered 12–48 hours after alcohol withdrawal. Occasionally they are the prelude to delirium tremens. The situation may be complicated by coexistent addition to and withdrawal of tranquillizers and related drugs. Focal features or an abnormal electroencephalogram (EEG) between seizures, suggest a pre-existing liability to epilepsy.

Movement Disorders

Recent reports implicate chronic alcoholism in the genesis of movement disorders. Carlen et al.[6] and Lang et al.[7] have described the provocation of Parkinsonism by alcohol withdrawal or chronic intoxication. The disease may have been brought to light by an effect of alcohol on the dopaminergic systems. Transient writhing movements may appear 9–10 days after alcohol withdrawal.[8]

Prolonged Alcohol Abuse

Wernicke's Encephalopathy

This frequently undiagnosed but treatable condition has an acute onset with the development of a triad of mental and behavioural changes, abnormal eye movements, and unsteadiness. Disorders of higher cerebral function occur in 90 per cent of cases. Most commonly this is a quiet global confusional state with apathy, disorientation, and disturbed memory function out of proportion to other cognitive deficits, sometimes with accompanying confabulation (making up false but plausible stories). Drowsiness is often evident, but stupor and coma are rare, being present in only 4 per cent and 1 per cent of cases respectively. Abnormal eye movements are present in most patients and include nystagmus and paralysis of the lateral rectus muscles.

The disorder may evolve over several days but its progress is promptly arrested by the intravenous administration of thiamine (vitamin B_1). In the series of Victor et al.[9] 17 per cent died in the acute stage; in the remainder, the global confusional state consistently recovered, at which stage memory difficulties became more obvious and persisted in 84 per cent as a typical Korsakoff's syndrome (see below). Paralysis of eye movements recovered within days or weeks but nystagmus frequently persisted. Loss of equilibrium recovered completely in 33 per cent, generally beginning within a few days of inception of treatment and sometimes continuing over the course of several months; it persisted in the remainder. It is possible that Wernicke's encephalopathy could be prevented if food or beverages were supplemented with thiamine (1.5 mg a day).

The autopsy study by Harper[10] from Perth, Australia, produced the unexpected finding that the diagnosis may be undetected in life in a disquietingly high proportion of individuals. Out of a total of fifty-one post-mortem examinations in which the changes of Wernicke's encephalopathy were found in the brain, only seven patients were known to have the condition during life. Some of these had died abruptly as the result of haemorrhagic brainstem lesions; epilepsy and hypothermia were other factors contributing to death.

Korsakoff's Syndrome

Korsakoff's psychosis may follow an acute episode of Wernicke's encephalopathy. Sometimes patients have features of Korsakoff's syndrome in association with ocular signs and unsteadiness but without an acute confusional state; yet others have never developed paralysis of eye movements or unsteadiness.[9]

Korsakoff's syndrome is characterized by a disproportionate impairment of memory in relation to other cognitive disturbances. It combines a retrograde amnesia (difficulty in recalling information acquired over a period of days, months, or years before the onset of the disorder) with difficulty in assimilating new information. Confabulation may be present but is inconsistent.

The overlap between Korsakoff's syndrome and Wernicke's encephalopathy indicates their common origin in thiamine deficiency. The acute syndrome is characterized pathologically by bilaterally symmetrical lesions in the diencephalon and brainstem, particularly in a periventricular distribution, while the changes in Korsakoff's syndrome differ only by being more chronic. The causes of Wernicke–Korsakoff syndrome may be multifactorial and not solely related to thiamine deficiency; there may be a direct effect of alcohol on nervous tissue and a deficiency of other vitamins.

Dementia

The concept of a generalized dementia related to alcoholism is still unsettled. The important distinction is from the memory-impaired Korsakoff's syndrome. Specific cognitive defects are demonstrable in chronic alcohol abusers with preserved general intelligence, especially in the context of persistent alcoholism, socioeconomic deprivation and resistance to rehabilitation. There is also suggestive evidence that chronic alcohol abuse, even in younger individuals, may lead to relatively mild and non-progressive intellectual impairment. Attempts to find a term other than 'alcoholic dementia', which has the connotation of a progressive disorder, have been unsuccessful. Evidence for intellectual deterioration is so far lacking, although there is unequivocal evidence from animal studies of nerve damage directly produced by chronic alcohol administration unrelated to vitamin deficiency.[11]

A further approach has been to assess the presence of cerebral atrophy by computerized tomographic (CT) scanning and magnetic resonance imaging (MRI). Such studies have shown clear evidence of loss of brain tissue, with both ventricular enlargement and sulcal widening.[12] An important feature is that there is a strong improvement in CT scan appearances with abstinence. MRI has so far yielded conflicting results as to cerebral water content in chronic alcoholic abusers[13] and the slow resolution appears to be too gradual to be entirely explained by restoration of a normal water and electrolyte content. Other mechanisms, such as regeneration of nerve cell proteins could be involved.[14] Loss of brain tissue, particularly the white matter rather than the cerebral cortex, is apparent after death in patients with chronic alcohol abuse; it is greater in those with Wernicke's encephalopathy and alcoholic liver disease.[15]

Cerebellar Degeneration

In some individuals, chronic alcohol abuse is associated with a gradually progressive cerebellar syndrome in the absence of paralysis of eye movements or memory difficulty.[5] Unsteadiness predominantly affects stance and gait, with little effect on the arms or on speech. Once established, the condition persists. Pathological changes are concentrated in the anterior and superior vermis but also affect the cerebellar hemispheres; their distribution resembles that encountered in Wernicke's encephalopathy. Alcoholic cerebellar degeneration is probably nutritional in origin.

Cerebrovascular Disease

Subdural and extradural haematoma (effusions of blood between the skull and the brain) are more frequent in excessive drinkers as a result of head injury. Excess alcohol consumption has been implicated in the occurrence of cerebral infarcts even in young adults.[16–18,25] The occurrence of strokes may be related to acute heavy bouts of drinking, possibly by influencing blood clotting,[19] or to hypertension (see p. 62). A link with subarachnoid haemorrhage has also been identified.[20]

Peripheral Nerve Damage

A symmetrical involvement of the distal sensory and motor nerves is a frequent complication of chronic alcohol abuse. It was encountered in about 10 per cent of patients admitted to Boston City Hospital.[5] It is relatively more common in women. Burning discomfort or pain in the feet and excessive skin sensitivity to touch may be troublesome. Weakness of the hip and thigh muscles is not unusual and hoarseness of the voice and difficulty in swallowing from degenerative changes in the nerves to the larynx may occur. Disturbances of sweating may also occur.

Alcoholic nerve damage occurs in relation to nutritional deprivation and the major aetiological factor is likely to be deficiency of thiamine and perhaps other B vitamins. The pathological changes, which consist of a distal axonal degeneration with secondary demyelination, resemble those of beri-beri. A contribution from a direct toxic effect by alcohol is not excluded.[21]

Excessive drinkers are prone to focal peripheral nerve lesions as a consequence of compression sustained when stuporose or during heavy sleep. 'Saturday night paralysis' of the arm due to compression of the radial nerve is the most familiar example.

Muscle Damage

Acute muscle damage causing pain, swelling, and weakness is a well-recognized complication of a prolonged heavy drinking bout.[22-25] The muscles of the upper part of the leg and arm are predominantly affected. Extensive destruction of muscle fibres leads to markedly elevated serum creatine kinase levels and myoglobinuria. Renal failure may result. With abstinence, complete recovery is usual in a matter of days or weeks, depending upon severity.

Chronic alcoholic muscle damage is common, but is reversible with abstinence. Many persistent heavy drinkers have weak and flabby muscles and often complain of a variety of symptoms such as low back pain and cramp in the calf muscles. Muscle fibre damage can be demonstrated microscopically and biochemically in about 60 per cent of these people.[24] Almost all of them show additional evidence of alcohol-related damage such as cirrhosis, poor nutrition, and peripheral nerve damage.

Continued alcohol consumption is accompanied by persistence and even deterioration of muscle damage. Abstinence, on the other hand, is associated with improvement in muscle function after three months and often with complete recovery within a year.

References

1. Urso, T., Gavaler, J.S., and Van Thiel, D.H. (1981) Blood Ethanol Levels in Sober Alcohol Users Seen in an Emergency Room. *Life Science* 28: 1053–056.
2. Mirsky, A., Piker, P., Rosenbaum, M., and Lederer, H. (1941) 'Adaptation' of Central Nervous System to Varying Concentrations of Alcohol in Blood. *Journal of the Study of Alcohol* 2: 35–45.
3. Le Blanc, A.E., Kalant, H., and Gibbins, R.J. (1975) Acute Tolerance to Ethanol in the Rat. *Psychopharmacologia* 41: 43–6.
4. Goodwin, D.W., Crane, J.B., and Guze, S.B. (1969) Alcoholic Blackouts: a Review and Clinical Study of 100 Alcoholics. *American Journal of Psychiatry* 126: 191–98.
5. Victor, M. and Adams, R.D. (1953) The Effect of Alcohol on the Nervous System. In *Metabolic and Toxic Diseases of the Nervous System. Research Publications of the Association for Research into Nervous and Mental Disorders* 32: 526–73.
6. Carlen, P.L., Lee, M.A., Jacob, M., and Livshits, O. (1981) Parkinsonism Provoked by Alcoholism. *Annals of Neurology* 9: 84–6.

7. Lang, A.E., Marsden, C.D., Obeso, J.A., and Parkes, J.D. (1982) Alcohol and Parkinson's Disease. *Annals of Neurology* 12: 254–56.
8. Fornazzari, L. and Carlen, P.L. (1982) Transient Choreiform Dyskinesias During Alcohol Withdrawal. *Canadian Journal of Neurological Science* 9: 89–90.
9. Victor, M., Adams, R., and Collins, G.H. (1971) *The Wernicke-Korsakoff Syndrome. A Clinical and Pathological Study of 245 Patients, 82 with Post-Mortem Examinations.* Oxford: Blackwell.
10. Harper, C. (1979) Wernicke's Encephalopathy: a More Common Disease than Realised. A Neuropathological Study of 51 Cases. *Journal of Neurology, Neurosurgery and Psychiatry* 42: 226–31.
11. Riley, J.N. and Walker D.W. (1978) Morphological Alterations in the Hippocampus after Long-Term Alcohol Consumption in Mice. *Science* 201: 646–48.
12. Bergman, H., Borg, S., Hindmarsh, T., Ideström, C.M., and Mützel, S. (1980) Computed Tomography of the Brain and Neuropsychological Assessment of Male Alcoholic Patients and a Random Sample from the General Male Population. *Acta Physiologica Scandinavica* 62: Suppl. 286, 77–88.
13. Smith, M.A., Chick, J., Kean, D.M., Douglas, R.H., Singer, A., Kendell, R.E., and Best, J.J. (1985) Brain Water in Chronic Alcoholic Patients Measured by Magnetic Resonance Imaging. *Lancet* 1: 1273–274.
14. Ron, M.A., Acker, W., Shaw, G.K., and Lishman, W.A. (1982) Computerized Tomography of the Brain in Chronic Alcoholism. *Brain* 105: 497–514.
15. Harper, C., and Kril, J. (1985) Brain Atrophy in Chronic Alcoholic Patients: a Quantitative Pathological Study. *Journal of Neurology, Neurosurgery and Psychiatry* 48: 211–17.
16. Hillbom, M. and Kaste, M. (1981) Ethanol Intoxication: a Risk Factor for Ischaemic Brain Infarction in Adolescents and Young Adults. *Stroke* 12: 422–25.
17. Lee, K. (1979) Alcoholism and Cerebrovascular Thrombosis in the Young. *Acta Neurologica Scandinavica* 59: 270–74.
18. Taylor, J.R. (1982) Alcohol and Strokes. *New England Journal of Medicine* 306: 1111.
19. Hillbom, M., Kaste, M., and Rasi, V. (1983) Can Ethanol Intoxication Affect Hemocoagulation to Increase the Risk of Brain Infarction in Young Adults? *Neurology* (Cleveland) 33: 381–84.
20. Hillbom, M. and Kaste, M. (1982) Alcohol Intoxication: a Risk Factor for Primary Subarachnoid Hemorrhage. *Neurology* (NY) 32: 706–11.
21. Behse, F. and Buchthal, F. (1977) Alcoholic Neuropathy: Clinical, Electro-physiological, and Biopsy Findings. *Annals of Neurology* 2: 95–110.
22. Ekbom, H., Hed, R., Kirstein, L., and Astrom, K. (1964) Muscular Affections in Chronic Alcoholism. *Archives of Neurology* (Chicago) 10: 449–58.
23. Perkoff, G.T., Hardy, P., and Velez-Garcia, E. (1966) Reversible Acute

Muscular Syndrome in Chronic Alcoholism. *New England Journal of Medicine* 274: 1277–284.
24. Martin, F., Ward, K., Slavin, G., Levi, J., and Peters, T.J. (1985) Alcoholic Skeletal Myopathy, a Clinical and Pathological Study. *Quarterly Journal of Medicine* 55: 233–51.
25. Gill, J.S., Zezulka, A.V., Shipley, M.J., Gill, S.K., and Beevers, D.G. (1986) Stroke and Alcohol Consumption. *New England Journal of Medicine* 315: 1041–046.

4

THE LIVER

Summary

Liver damage is common in patients drinking excessive amounts of alcohol. The majority will develop fatty change in the liver, but 10–30 per cent will eventually develop cirrhosis. Early liver lesions will heal if drinking ceases and individuals with cirrhosis will live longer if they abstain. Liver cancer develops as a late complication of cirrhosis in approximately 10 per cent of patients.

Excess alcohol consumption leads to the development of a wide range of liver injury and although cirrhosis is the most serious form, it develops in less than one-third of heavy drinkers.[1,2]

The clinical spectrum of alcoholic liver disease extends from symptomless enlargement of the liver (hepatomegaly) to liver failure with jaundice, fluid in the abdomen (ascites), and bleeding from the gut. Clinical signs and laboratory tests cannot be relied upon to differentiate the various stages of alcoholic liver disease; patients with precirrhotic disease may show severe liver failure while those with well-compensated cirrhosis may have no symptoms and show few abnormalities in laboratory tests. Liver biopsy examination is mandatory for diagnosis.

Fatty Liver

Most alcohol abusers will develop fatty change in the liver at some stage of their drinking career. Although fat accumulation indicates a profound metabolic disturbance within the liver, it is not necessarily harmful.[3] The majority of patients with simple fatty liver have no symptoms, although some complain of pain on the right side of the upper abdomen or non-specific digestive problems such as nausea, loss of appetite, epigastric discomfort, or bowel disturbances. Hepatomegaly is the most common sign: the liver is smooth and only mildly tender; the liver edge is regular and may extend a few centimetres below the rib margin or low into the right abdomen. Other frequent physical findings include dilated blood vessels in the skin (spider naevi), reddening of the palms of the hands (palmar erythema), parotid gland swelling, and tendon contractions in the hand (Dupuytren's contractures). The most common biochemical abnormalities are increased values of the serum enzymes, aspartate aminotransferase (AST) and gamma-glutamyl transferase (GGT); abnormally large red blood cells (macrocytes) are usually present. Liver biopsy shows mild to severe fat accumulation in the liver cell.

Alcoholic Hepatitis

Alcoholic hepatitis develops in only a proportion of heavy drinkers even after decades of drinking.[4] The cell destruction observed in the liver when this lesion is present may play an important role in the development of cirrhosis. However, in 52 per cent of patients, alcoholic hepatitis persists unchanged for several years and in 10 per cent it may heal despite continued alcohol abuse,[5] suggesting that other mechanisms play an important role in the progression of the liver injury.

Alcoholic hepatitis may vary in its presentation from a mild illness without jaundice to a serious and often fatal disorder with jaundice, ascites, gastro-intestinal bleeding and hepatic coma. The majority of patients complain of loss of appetite, malaise, fatigue, and pain on the right side of the abdomen. Patients are often feverish and malnourished. Spider naevi, palmar erythema, and bruising of the skin are prominent; wound healing is generally poor. The liver is usually moderately enlarged and tender and there may be an audible arterial bruit over it. Enlargement of the spleen and other features of increased pressure in the portal blood vessels are seen in some patients. Frank failure of liver cell function may be present. Kidney failure develops shortly before death in a high proportion of the more severely ill patients. Serum levels of AST and GGT are generally higher than in other forms of alcohol-related liver disease. Serum alkaline phosphatase values are often elevated and serum bilirubin values may appear disproportionately high. Anaemia and macrocytosis are common; there is an increase in the number of circulating white blood cells in all but the mildest cases. Blood clotting is disturbed as shown by low platelet counts and prolonged prothrombin times which are incompletely reversed by injections of vitamin K_1. Liver biopsy reveals a predominantly centrizonal lesion with liver cell swelling, inflammatory infiltrates, pericellular fibrosis, and varying degrees of cell death and accumulation of fat and bile pigment. Mallory's alcoholic hyaline, if centrally distributed, is considered diagnostic of this lesion. Patients with alcoholic hepatitis are generally more ill than patients with simple fatty liver.

Cirrhosis

Patients with well-compensated cirrhosis may have no symptoms or complain only of loss of appetite and fatigue. Patients with decompensated cirrhosis show features of liver cell failure such as jaundice, ascites, oedema of the legs, and of increased pressure in the portal vein which manifests as haemorrhage from distended oesophageal veins. Episodic or persistent neuropsychiatric changes secondary to a metabolic disturbance of the brain may be present. Spider naevi, palmar erythema, and a low grade fever are commonly found. The liver is usually enlarged, but enlargement of the spleen is only observed in 25 per cent of patients. Serum enzymes are usually only moderately elevated; the concentration of bilirubin in the blood varies with the degree of decompensation. Macrocytosis is common and the prothrombin time is usually prolonged. Liver biopsy generally shows a micronodular cirrhosis though macronodular change is more commonly observed in abstinent patients. Varying degrees of fatty infiltration and/or alcoholic hepatitis may be seen within cirrhotic nodules in actively drinking subjects.

Primary Liver Cell Cancer

In Britain primary liver cell cancer develops in between 3 and 11 per cent of individuals with alcoholic cirrhosis.[6–8] It occurs three times more often in men than in women and is more likely to develop in patients who have been abstinent from alcohol in later life than in those who continue to drink.[9] In one-third of the patients who die with alcoholic cirrhosis, death can be attributed to the development of primary liver cell cancer.[6,7]

Primary liver cell cancer should be suspected if a patient with alcoholic cirrhosis develops abdominal pain, increasing resistance to diuretic drugs, sudden deterioration in liver function tests, or increasing enlargement of the liver. Patients may, however, present suddenly with uncontrollable bleeding from the gut.[10]

Fifty per cent of patients with alcoholic cirrhosis who develop primary liver cell cancer show increased plasma levels of alpha-fetoprotein. The diagnosis rests on the demonstration of an abnormal blood circulation pattern within the liver and histological proof on liver biopsy.

Susceptibility to Liver Damage

An individual's susceptibility to alcohol-related liver injury is probably determined by a number of genetic,[11] constitutional and environmental factors. Several studies have suggested that women are more susceptible to the hepatotoxic effects of alcohol than men.[6] Following a standard oral dose of alcohol women achieve significantly higher plasma alcohol concentrations than men because their total body water is smaller.[12] Tissue alcohol concentrations are correspondingly higher and it is reasonable to suppose that over a period of time this might result in earlier or more severe tissue damage. Several studies point to a relationship between the potential to develop alcoholic cirrhosis and the presence of certain HLA tissue types. There is a weak association between alcoholic cirrhosis and the presence of tissue antigens Aw32, B8, B13, B27, and B37.[13] The presence of HLA B8 in particular may influence the rate at which cirrhosis develops and the nature of the pre-cirrhotic lesion.[14,15] Ethnic origin may also be important; in the United States the age-adjusted incidence rates for alcoholic liver disease are substantially higher in the black population.[16]

Many attempts have been made to study the quantitative relationship between daily alcohol consumption and the risk of developing alcoholic liver disease. In the earliest studies, Lelbach[17–19] determined that there was a logarithmic correlation between the cumulative consumption of alcohol in relation to body weight and the relative frequency of severe liver damage. The risk increased sharply for a 70 kg man drinking 6 units a day (50 g) for ten years. Following this, a series of studies were carried out in France, which were based on results of dietary interviews carried out by specially trained dieticians. Péquignot[20,21] found that in men the relative risk of cirrhosis was six times greater at 5–7.5 units a day (40–60 g) than at 0–2.5 units a day (0–20 g) and 14 times greater at 7.5–10 units a day (60–80 g). The risk in women, however, began to increase with daily alcohol intakes of over 2.5 units (20 g). Because of the design of Péquignot's studies, no comment can be made regarding the time period of consumption necessary to produce damage. It has also been suggested recently that Péquignot may actually have under-estimated consumption in the cirrhotic patients.[22] Durbec et al. also

found a direct correlation between the logarithm of the relative risk
of cirrhosis and mean daily alcohol consumption up to intakes of
22.5 units (180 g).[23] Beyond this level they found no further
augmentation of risk in men.

Two recent case control studies have been carried out in Toronto
to investigate the risk of fatty infiltration and cirrhosis of the liver
in men and women in relation to varying levels of alcohol
consumption.[24,25] Men drinking about 5 units (40 g) alcohol a day
are nearly six times more likely to develop fatty livers than non-
drinkers, and this chance increases to sixty times in those drinking
more than 10 units (80 g) daily. For cirrhosis of the liver, the odds
are twice as great for the first group and rise to 117 for the heavier
drinkers. In women, the chance of developing fatty liver is nearly
three times as great at only 2.5 units (20 g) a day, rising to nine times
with drinking more than 7.5 units (60 g) daily; for cirrhosis the
figures at these levels of drinking are 2.5 and 14 respectively.

However, it is important to emphasize that such attempts to define
a threshold of hazardous consumption lead only to statistical average
values and that these may have little validity for a given individual
because of the wide variability in the susceptibility to damage.

The relationship between malnutrition and alcoholic liver injury is
discussed in Chapter 6.

Management of Alcoholic Liver Disease

The most effective treatment for alcoholic liver disease is abstinence
from alcohol. Patients with fatty liver should be advised to abstain
and take a balanced diet; no further measures are required. Patients
with alcoholic hepatitis require bed rest in hospital and intensive
nutritional support; abstinence from alcohol is mandatory. Complications such as infection, gastro-intestinal bleeding, mental
damage, and fluid retention require skilled attention. Corticosteroids
generally confer no benefit. Patients with well-compensated cirrhosis
must also abstain from alcohol and take a well-balanced diet; no
further measures will be required. Decompensated liver disease
requires experienced management and nutritional support.

Prognosis

Prognosis is determined to a large extent by the subsequent drinking
behaviour: with fatty liver it is excellent if patients subsequently
abstain. Alcoholic hepatitis, on the other hand, carries a significant

mortality: in patients ill enough to need admission to hospital but well enough for liver biopsy to be performed, the mortality ranges from 1.5–8.0 per cent.[26,27] In patients with severe, uncorrectable clotting abnormalities, it is nearer 60 per cent. The prognosis depends largely on the severity of the initial illness but long-term survival is significantly improved by the discontinuation or reduction of alcohol consumption. Patients with alcoholic hepatitis who reduce their alcohol intake, have an 80 per cent seven-year survival compared with a 50 per cent seven-year survival in those who continue to drink.[28] Survival in patients with alcoholic cirrhosis is significantly improved with abstinence even in those with decompensated disease.[7] Individuals who develop primary liver cell cancer are unlikely to survive beyond six months.

References

1. Lelbach, W.K. (1966) Leberschaden bei chronischem Alkoholismus I–II. *Acta Hepatosplenologica* 13: 321–49.
2. Leevy, C.M. (1968) Cirrhosis in Alcoholics. *Medical Clinics of North America* 52: 1445–451.
3. Lieber, C.S. (1975) Liver Disease and Alcohol: Fatty Liver, Alcoholic Hepatitis, Cirrhosis and their Interrelationships. *Annals of the New York Academy of Sciences* 252: 63–84.
4. Lelbach, W.K. (1975) Cirrhosis in the Alcoholic and its Relation to the Volume of Alcohol Abuse. *Annals of the New York Academy of Sciences* 252: 85–105.
5. Galambos, J.T. (1972) Natural History of Alcoholic Hepatitis. III. Histological Change. *Gastroenterology* 63: 1026–035.
6. Morgan, M.Y. and Sherlock, S. (1977) Sex-Related Differences Among 100 Patients with Alcoholic Liver Disease. *British Medical Journal* i: 939–41.
7. Saunders, J.B., Walters, J.R.F., Davies, P., and Paton, A. (1981) A 20 Year Prospective Study of Cirrhosis. *British Medical Journal* 282: 263–66.
8. Morgan, M.Y. (1984) Epidemiology of Alcoholic Liver Disease: United Kingdom. In P. Hall (ed.) *Alcoholic Liver Disease*. London: Edward Arnold, pp. 193–229.
9. Lee, F.I. (1966) Cirrhosis and Hepatoma in Alcoholics. *Gut* 7: 77–85.
10. Stone, W.D., Islam, N.R.K., and Paton, A. (1968) The Natural History of Cirrhosis. Experience with an Unselected Group of Patients. *Quarterly Journal of Medicine* 37: 119–32.
11. Saunders, J.B. and Williams, R. (1983) The Genetics of Alcoholism: is there an Inherited Susceptibility to Alcohol-Related Problems? *Alcohol and Alcoholism* 18: 189–217.
12. Marshall, A.W., Kingstone, D., Boss, A.M., and Morgan, M.Y. (1983) Ethanol Elimination in Males and Females: Relationship to Menstrual

Cycle and Body Composition. *Hepatology* 3: 701–06.
13. Eddleston, A.L.W.F. and Davis, M. (1982) Histocompatibility Antigens in Alcoholic Liver Disease. *British Medical Bulletin* 38: 13–16.
14. Morgan, M.Y., Ross, M.G.R., Ng, C.M., Adams, D.M., Thomas, H.C., and Sherlock, S. (1980) HLA-B8, Immunoglobulins, and Antibody Responses in Alcohol-Related Liver Disease. *Journal of Clinical Pathology* 33: 488–92.
15. Saunders, J.B., Haines, A., Portmann, B., Wodak, A.D., Powell-Jackson, P.R., Davis, M., and Williams, R. (1982) Accelerated Development of Alcoholic Cirrhosis in Patients with HLA-B8. *Lancet* 1: 1381–384.
16. Gargaliano, C.F., Mendeloff, A.I., and Lilienfeld, A.M. (1977) Incidence of Liver Cirrhosis in 16 Areas of the US. *Gastroenterology* 72: 1060.
17. Lelbach, W.K. (1972) Dosis-Wirkungs-Beziehung bei Alkohol-Leberschaden. *Deutsche Medizinische Wochenschrift* 97: 1435–436.
18. Lelbach, W.K. (1975) Quantitative Aspects of Drinking in Alcoholic Liver Cirrhosis. In J. M. Khanna, Y. Israel, and H. Kalant (eds) *Alcoholic Liver Pathology*. Toronto: Addiction Research Foundation, pp. 1–18.
19. Lelbach, W.K. (1985) Epidemiology of Alcoholic Liver Disease: Continental Europe. In P. Hall (ed.) *Alcoholic Liver Disease. Pathobiology, Epidemiology and Clinical Aspects*. London: Edward Arnold, pp. 130–66.
20. Péquignot, G., Chabert, C., Eydoux, H., and Courcoul, M.A. (1974) Augmentation du Risque de Cirrhose en Fonction de la Ration d'Alcool. *Revue de L'Alcool* 20: 191–202.
21. Péquignot, G., Tuyns, A.G., and Berta, J.L. (1978) Ascitic Cirrhosis in Relation to Alcohol Consumption. *International Journal of Epidemiology* 7: 113–20.
22. Chick, J. (1982) Epidemiology of Alcohol Use and its Hazards. *British Medical Bulletin* 38: 3–8.
23. Durbec, J.P., Bidart, J.M., and Sarles, H. (1979) Etude des Variations du Risque de Cirrhose du Foie en Fonction de la Consommation d'Alcool. *Gastroentérologie Clinique et Biologique* 3: 725–44.
24. Coates, R.A., Halliday, M.L., Rankin, J.G., Feinman, S.V., and Fisher, M.M. (1984) Risk of Fatty Infiltration to Ethanol Consumption: a Case-Control Study. *Hepatology* 4: 1015.
25. Coates, R.A., Halliday, M.L., Rankin, J.G., Feinman, S.V., and Fisher, M.M. (1984) A Case-Control Study of the Risk of Cirrhosis of the Liver in Relation to Ethanol Consumption. *Hepatology* 4: 1015.
26. Green, J., Mistilis, S., and Schiff, L. (1963) Acute Alcoholic Hepatitis. *Archives of Internal Medicine* 112: 67–78.
27. Lischner, M.W., Alexander, J.F., and Galambos, J.T. (1971) Natural History of Alcoholic Hepatitis. I. The Acute Disease. *American Journal of Digestive Diseases* 16: 481–94.
28. Galambos, J.T. (1974) Alcoholic Hepatitis. In F. Schaffner, S. Sherlock and C. M. Leevy (eds) *The Liver and its Diseases*. New York: Intercontinental Medical Books, pp. 255–67.

5

THE GASTRO-INTESTINAL
SYSTEM AND PANCREAS

Summary

The most important effects of alcohol on the gut are the predisposition to cancer of the oesophagus and the precipitation of acute and chronic pancreatitis, which may cause intermittent or protracted pain, together with endocrine and exocrine failure. Less dangerous but disabling are the nausea and retching due to alcoholic gastritis.

Oesophagus

Alcohol increases gastro-oesophageal reflux and healing of reflux oesophagitis is more likely to occur if alcohol is withdrawn.[1] The Mallory–Weiss syndrome is a laceration of the mucosa at the gastro-oesophageal junction giving rise to bleeding and about 40 per cent of such patients are abusing alcohol which induces the nausea and vomiting.[2] Rarely the tear is so deep as to cause rupture of the oesophagus with consequent inflammation of the tissues surrounding it. The most dangerous oesophageal consequence of alcohol abuse is cancer of the oesophagus which has a five-year survival rarely greater than 5 per cent. The incidence of cancer of the oesophagus in Europe is greatest in France and the varying rates in that country are proportional to alcohol intake.[3] Religious groups in a high incidence area who do not take alcohol are much less affected by oesophageal cancer.[4] The alcohol effect is potentiated by tobacco and it has been estimated that the risk of developing cancer of the oesophagus is increased eighteen-fold in those who drink more than ten units

(80 g) of alcohol a day and by a factor of forty-four when, in addition, they smoke twenty cigarettes a day.[5]

Stomach

Alcohol causes acute gastritis which heals within a few days of abstinence. It is thought to account for the typical early morning nausea and retching of alcohol abuse and possibly bleeding from gastric erosions; it does not proceed to permanent damage of the mucosa. Although it has been stated that alcohol causes gastric or duodenal ulcers, there is no evidence to support this contention; it may, however, aggravate them or impair healing.

Intestine

Diarrhoea may be the presenting clinical complaint of the alcohol abuser. Alcohol has been shown to inhibit many transport processes in the small gut mucosa, but the importance of these in the development of malnutrition in the alcohol abuser is debatable and it seems that decreased intake and interference with metabolism are more important[6] (see Chapter 6).

Pancreas

Alcohol is an important cause of chronic pancreatitis in Western cultures in at least 50 per cent of patients.[7] There is a direct correlation between consumption of alcohol and the risk of developing chronic pancreatitis. In one survey, when daily consumption of alcohol was recorded and the patients divided into groups at 3 units (20 g) per day intervals, there was a significant correlation between daily consumption and the logarithm of the risk. This indicates that there is no single threshold of toxicity but probably a continuous variation of thresholds between individuals, so that some people must be assumed to be exquisitely sensitive.[8] In Copenhagen the frequency of chronic pancreatitis has increased together with the increased consumption of alcohol.[9] Long continuous abuse is important in the genesis of clinically significant damage, the mean time being 10–12 years for women and 17–18 years for men.[8]

The dominant clinical feature of chronic pancreatitis is pain. The initial attacks are clinically indistinguishable from acute pancreatitis but take place in a gland already damaged. When the pain resolves, the damage persists and progresses. Pain occurs in 60–100 per cent of patients and can be so disabling as to need morphine-related analgesics, although the intensity tends to decline over the years. Complications of the acute attacks are false cysts which may leak, causing splenic vein block, and protracted obstructive jaundice from pressure on the common bile duct in the head of the pancreas. Transient jaundice may result from oedema of the head of the pancreas.

The two main effects of chronic destruction of the pancreas are failure of pancreatic hormone-secreting cells causing diabetes mellitus, and failure of the enzyme-secreting cells causing maldigestion of food and so malabsorption and malnutrition. Diabetes occurs in approximately half the patients,[9] 50 per cent of whom need insulin. The diabetes is often difficult to control and periods of low blood sugar are common. Such patients may develop all the complications of diabetes mellitus. Deficiency of secretion of digestive enzymes causing excess fat excretion also occurs in over 50 per cent of patients. In some series there is a high incidence of carcinoma of the pancreas.[9] The prognosis of chronic pancreatitis is poor, whether or not the patients undergo operative treatment for pain; the ten-year survival is less than 50 per cent,[10,11] half the deaths being due to pancreatic causes and the other half to other alcohol-related disorders.[12]

References

1. Weinbeck, M. and Berges, W. (1981) Oesophageal Lesions in the Alcoholic. *Clinics in Gastroenterology* 10: 375–88.
2. Knauer, C.M. (1976) Mallory–Weiss Syndrome. *Gastroenterology* 71: 5–8.
3. Audigier, J.C., Tuyns, A.J., and Lambert, R. (1975) Epidemiology of Oesophageal Cancer in France: Increasing Mortality and Persistent Correlation with Alcoholism. *Digestion* 13: 209–19.
4. Enstrom, J.E. (1978) Cancer Mortality Among Normans. *Cancer* 36: 835–41.
5. Tuyns, A.J., Péquignot, G., and Jensen, O.M. (1977) Le Cancer de l'Oesophage en Ille-et-Vilaine en Fonction des Niveaux de Consommation d'Alcool et de Tabac. *Bulletin du Cancer* 64: 45–60.
6. Gazzard, B.G. and Clark, M. (1978) Alcohol and the Alimentary System. *Clinical Endocrinology and Metabolism* 7: 429–45.
7. Worning, H. (1984) Chronic Pancreatitis: Pathogenesis, Natural History and Conservative Treatment. *Clinical Gastroenterology* 13: 871–94.
8. Durbec, J.P. and Sarles, H. (1978) Multicentre Survey of the Aetiology of Pancreatic Disease. *Digestion* 18: 337–50.

9. Anderson, B.N., Pedersen, N.T., Scheel, J., and Worning, H. (1982) Incidence of Alcoholic Chronic Pancreatitis in Copenhagen. *Scandinavian Journal of Gastroenterology* 17: 247–52.

10. Pedersen, N.T., Anderson, B.N., Pedersen, G., and Worning, H. (1982) Chronic Pancreatitis in Copenhagen. *Scandinavian Journal of Gastroenterology* 17: 925–31.

11. White, T.T. and Slavotinek, A.H. (1979) Results of Surgical Treatment of Chronic Pancreatitis. *Annals of Surgery* 189: 217–24.

12. Strum, W.B. and Spiro, H.M. (1971) Chronic Pancreatitis. *Annals of International Medicine* 74: 264–77.

6

NUTRITION

Summary

The cumulative toxic effects of alcohol and the accompanying malnutrition involve many of the body's organs. There is progressive brain and liver damage and the body's defence mechanisms become increasingly unable to withstand the continued attacks from infections and other stresses.

Alcohol abuse is commonly associated with malnutrition.[1] The single most important factor is inadequate intake of most foods, especially protein, but the contributions made by the toxic effects of alcohol on the gastro-intestinal tract, impaired utilization of nutrients, and their excessive loss, play an increasing part in the progressive deterioration.[2]

The diagnosis of generalized malnutrition lies at an arbitrary point on a curve relating functional loss to increasing nutritional impairment. There is no cut-off point, only an accumulating inefficiency and a reduced capability for coping with further injury.[3]

In order to achieve good nutrition an adequate supply of carbohydrate, fat, and protein, together with essential vitamins and minerals, is necessary for energy metabolism and synthetic processes, to support growth and effect repair of damaged tissues. Failure of an adequate supply of either or both groups of these substances constitutes malnutrition. Malnutrition usually predates significant brain and liver damage.[4]

Evidence of Malnutrition

One gram of alcohol supplies 7.1 kilocalories of energy and one litre of spirits contains approximately 2300 kilocalories. Since the liver preferentially metabolizes alcohol and because alcoholic beverages contain only small amounts of nutrients which are inadequate to

meet daily requirements, the 'empty' calories derived from alcohol
make no contribution to nutrition other than energy; under some
circumstances this will result in obesity. It is for this reason that
obesity may be seen in the early stages of heavy drinking.[5]

More commonly, however, alcohol-associated malnutrition results
in weight loss.[2] The alcohol content of the diet causes an imbalance
in terms of energy derived from other sources such as fat and
protein; they become increasingly deficient as the alcohol content is
increased, usually to the exclusion of high quality protein (*Figure 5*).
This dietary imbalance may increase the demand for specific
nutrients, particularly vitamins. Thiamine deficiency has been
reported in 30–80 per cent of alcohol abusers, folic acid deficiency in
6–80 per cent, and low levels of pyridoxine have been seen in 50 per
cent. Nicotinic acid and vitamin B_{12} deficiencies are much less
frequent.[6]

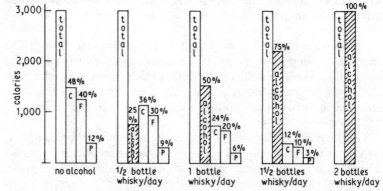

Figure 5 The effect of isocaloric replacement of dietary constituents by
alcohol on the overall consumption of the caloric intake. For a fixed daily
intake of 3000 calories the effect of increasing dietary substitution with
alcohol on the proportion of total calories derived from the remaining
carbohydrate (C), fat (F), and protein (P) in the diet is shown. (Reproduced
by kind permission of *Alcohol and Alcoholism*.[2])

Causes of Malnutrition

The body weight of middle-class excessive drinkers may meet, or
even exceed, their ideal weight. Although their nutrient intake when
judged by recall histories, appears to satisfy recommended daily
allowances for non-drinking individuals, energy intake from protein,
fat, and carbohydrate is often reduced or imbalanced because of the
alcohol load. As the condition progresses and the social consequences of

drinking begin to have their influence, limited funds are often used to buy alcohol rather than food. Large doses of alcohol depress hunger and habits such as excessive cigarette smoking and coffee drinking, together with the gastro-intestinal and metabolic effects of alcohol, contribute to the malnutrition (*Table* 7).

Table 7 *Factors contributing to malnutrition*

Reduced total food intake.
Imbalance between dietary constituents.
Impaired digestion and absorption of food.
Increased nutrient requirements.
Inadequate tissue storage of nutrients.
Impaired nutrient utilization.
Increased urinary and faecal losses.

Consequences of Malnutrition

Malnutrition itself plays an important part in producing changes in body composition and causing damage to the liver and the nervous system.

Changes in body composition

Chronic excessive alcohol consumption is generally associated with weight loss: thus either abstinence from alcohol or improvement in the diet could account for the observed weight gain following admission to hospital. However, it is likely that improved food intake is the major factor since, when 56 excessive drinkers were admitted to hospital and were given a normal diet (2600 Kcal), no additional weight gain was observed in 17 who received a further 1800 Kcals each day as alcohol (256 grams).[7] Similarly, under experimental conditions, 11 normal subjects lost weight when half their total calories taken as carbohydrate were gradually replaced by alcohol. In the same study, the addition of 2000 Kcals daily as alcohol to the diet of one alcohol abuser produced no consistent change in body weight, whereas the addition of 2000 Kcals daily as chocolate resulted in consistent weight gain (*Figure* 6).[7]

   These observations suggest that the calorie supply from alcohol is largely offset by other dietary, endocrine, or metabolic factors associated with high alcohol consumption. The metabolic response to alcohol in excessive drinkers differs from that in people who drink

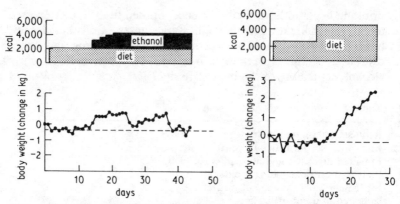

Figure 6 (a) The effect on body weight of adding 2000 Kcal/day as ethanol
to the diet of one subject. The dotted line represents the mean change
during the control period. (b) The effect on body weight of adding
2000 Kcal/day as chocolate to the diet of the same subject as in Figure 6(a).
The dotted line represents the mean change during the control period.
(Data from Pirolä and Lieber,[7] reproduced by kind permission of *Alcohol
and Alcoholism.*)

within safe limits: in the former there is a much greater increase in
oxygen consumption after a single large dose of alcohol. This 'energy
wastage' helps to explain the weight loss observed in subjects
drinking excessively, but its mechanism is unknown.

Even before weight loss occurs, there is evidence that body
composition changes; when weight begins to fall, body fat starts to
disappear and there is wasting of muscles. Less apparent is the loss
in mineral content of bones. The combined effect of reduced energy
provision and reduced nutrient intake is partial starvation. Alcohol
impairs glucose synthesis by the liver while accelerating the
breakdown of glycogen and exhausting muscle glycogen stores.
Muscle breakdown also results in loss of magnesium, zinc, and
nitrogen in the urine. The falling blood glucose level results in
increased breakdown of fat to fatty acids; these are then, in part,
oxidized in the liver and, in part, converted to ketone bodies which
can be used as energy by brain, heart, and muscles.

Liver Injury

Most workers today would accept that both malnutrition and alcohol
toxicity play an important part in damaging the liver but would
probably disagree about the relative contribution each of them

makes. When protein deficiency is present it may potentiate the effect of alcohol but, because alcohol itself plays a key role in the development of liver injury, heavy drinkers, even if they do attempt to maintain a high protein diet, would not succeed in preventing the development of cirrhosis unless they also reduce their alcohol intake. Patients with alcoholic cirrhosis develop the catabolic state of starvation more readily than normal individuals and the metabolic reactions required to maintain a stable fuel supply to the body's essential organs, such as the heart and brain, may partly explain the severe wasting of some patients. It is important to recognize the existence of malnutrition because its correction by appropriate therapy, together with reduced alcohol intake, has been reported to increase survival and accelerate improvement in patients with alcohol-related liver injury.[4]

Central Nervous System Damage

Alcohol itself causes some structural alterations in brain tissue. In addition, chronic alcohol abusers exhibit a number of neurological disorders which are directly related to nutritional deficiencies.[8] Vitamin deficiencies are of particular importance, especially thiamine, nicotinic acid, pyridoxine, and vitamin B_{12}, all of which are essential for normal cerebral functioning. Marginal deficiencies produce alterations in behaviour while more severe deprivation over a period of time may produce irreversible structural cerebral changes. Clinical and laboratory evidence shows that chronic alcohol abuse is accompanied by a reduction in both total body and available circulating thiamine. The typical Wernicke–Korsakoff syndrome due to thiamine deficiency develops only in a minority of subjects but is much more frequently present, and sometimes unrecognized, in a milder form which is characterized by changes in affect, considered judgement, and memory (see Chapter 3). Differences in the activity of the thiamine-dependent enzyme transketolase may explain why some individuals are particularly at risk of brain damage.[9]

Malabsorption may also cause other vitamin deficiencies: nicotinic acid deficiency (combined with low tryptophan intake) results in pellagra, diarrhoea, dermatitis, and dementia, and pyridoxine deficiency can produce both behavioural and electrophysiological changes. There is some evidence that alcohol may, by enhancing certain enzymes outside the nervous system, divert the available vitamins away from the brain.

Nutritional Replacement

Since vitamin deficiencies are relatively common in individuals who drink excessively, extra vitamins are frequently given without determining whether deficiencies are present. Supplementation needs to be in a form which can be absorbed from the gut or can be given by injection to guarantee that it will reach the tissues. Such an approach is acceptable for some water-soluble vitamins, excess of which is not usually associated with toxicity, although pyridoxine toxicity has been described. Care must be taken with the fat-soluble vitamin A because an excess may, in itself, cause liver injury.

The optimal form of nutritional therapy and its potential benefit at early stages of alcohol damage remains to be documented. However, even when complications of cirrhosis are present, nutritional intervention can improve impaired brain function.

References

1. Thomson, A.D., Rae, S.A., and Majumdar, S.K. (1980) Malnutrition in the Alcoholic. In P. M. S. Clarke and L. J. Kricka (eds) *Medical Consequences of Alcohol Abuse*. Chichester: Ellis Horwood, pp. 103–55.
2. World, M.J., Ryle, P.R., and Thomson, A.D. (1985) Alcoholic Malnutrition and the Small Intestine. *Alcohol and Alcoholism* 20: 89–124.
3. World, M.J., Ryle, P.R., Jones, D., Shaw, G.K., and Thomson, A.D. (1984) Differential Effect of Chronic Alcohol Intake and Poor Malnutrition on Bodyweight and Fat Stores. *Alcohol and Alcoholism* 19: 281–90.
4. Mendenhall, C.L., Anderson, S., Weesner, R.E., Goldberg, S.J., and Crolic, K. A. (1984) Protein-Calorie Malnutrition Associated with Alcoholic Hepatitis. *American Journal of Medicine* 76: 211–22.
5. Sherlock, S. (1984) Nutrition and the Alcoholic. *Lancet* I: 436–38.
6. Morgan, M.Y. (1982) Alcohol and Nutrition. *British Medical Bulletin* 38: 21–9.
7. Pirolä, R.C. and Lieber, C.S. (1972) The Energy Cost of the Metabolism of Drugs, Including Ethanol. *Pharmacology* 7: 185–96.
8. Thomson, A.D., Ryle, P.R., and Shaw, G.K. (1983) Ethanol, Thiamine and Brain Damage. *Alcohol and Alcoholism* 18: 27–43.
9. Pratt, O.E., Jeyasingham, M., Shaw, G.K., and Thomson, A.D. (1985) Transketolase Variant Enzymes and Brain Damage. *Alcohol and Alcoholism* 20: 223–32.

7

HEART DISEASE

Summary

Alcohol reduces the strength of the heart beat and can precipitate irregularities in its rhythm. These rhythm disturbances usually follow binge drinking and do not presage chronic heart disease. Continuing alcohol excess may contribute to permanent failure of the heart and anyone with failing heart muscle should be advised not to drink alcohol. Alcohol itself is not a risk factor for coronary heart disease.

Disease of the Heart Muscle

Alcohol may cause damage to the heart muscle (cardiomyopathy) by three different mechanisms:

1. A direct toxic effect of alcohol and its metabolites on the metabolism of the heart muscle cell.[1]
2. Associated nutritional defects, particularly deficiency of thiamine.
3. Toxic effects due to additives such as cobalt.

Direct effects of alcohol

Acute effects

Acute administration of alcohol results in depression of the force of contraction of the heart muscle with temporary reduction in the volume of blood ejected from the left ventricle. This is more marked in non-drinkers than in otherwise fit subjects who are habituated to alcohol. Conversely, the chronic alcohol abuser with myocardial dysfunction is more susceptible to the effects of an acute challenge with alcohol than the normal individual.[2] Binge drinking can produce abnormal heart rhythms such as paroxysmal atrial fibrillation, ventricular ectopic beats, or ventricular tachycardia. This has been

termed 'the holiday heart' syndrome.[3] Sufferers have no other
evidence of heart disease and the irregularity disappears without
residue, though moderate conduction delays have been noted when
these patients are assessed by high-speed electrocardiography a week
after restoration of normal sinus rhythm. These events do not
presage the development of chronic cardiomyopathy.[2]

Apparently healthy individuals may sometimes develop abnormal
rhythms after even modest quantities of alcohol, and chronic alcohol
abuse may cause slow atrial fibrillation.

Alcohol can induce myocardial dysfunction even when adequate
nutrition is ensured. In one US study a well-nourished alcohol
abuser was given 12–16 units of whisky (96–128 g alcohol) daily for
several months and developed gradual (though mild) heart failure
which disappeared within several weeks of cessation of alcohol
without other specific therapy.[4]

Cardiomyopathy

'Excessive consumption of alcohol is the major cause of secondary,
non-ischaemic, dilated cardiomyopathy in the Western World'.[5]
This is an extreme view but it is popularly believed that alcoholic
cardiomyopathy is a distinct condition caused by excessive consumption of alcohol.[6] Others think that alcohol may play a
conditioning or precipitating role.[7] At present one cannot distinguish a
causal versus conditioning role nor apply precise criteria to its
diagnosis. Furthermore the clinical, laboratory, and pathological
appearances of alcoholic cardiomyopathy do not differ from those of
non-alcoholic dilated cardiomyopathy.

Alcohol may be one of several contributory causes to dilated
cardiomyopathy. Cardiac reserves are large and we know little of the
frequency of subclinical myocardial malfunction and its causes.
Increased alcohol intake might precipitate symptoms of heart
failure, but an acute viral infection of the heart muscle might do the
same. Chronic alcohol consumption might lead to a state of
continued myocardial depression which is initially reversible through
abstention from alcohol but eventually becomes progressive. Progression and irreversibility become certain once the left ventricle has
dilated beyond a certain point. It is therefore prudent to advise all
patients with dilated cardiomyopathy to abstain permanently from
alcohol. Complete abstinence from alcohol is mandatory not only for
patients with alcoholic heart damage but also in those with dilated
cardiomyopathy from other causes because alcohol is a drug which is
bad for bad hearts. Eighty per cent of individuals with alcoholic

cardiomyopathy who continue to drink are dead within three years of diagnosis. A much quoted, small study from Chicago in excessively drinking non-smokers showed that total abstinence was followed by an 80 per cent long-term survival; a great improvement on what was expected, although not all patients who abstained did well.[8]

The incidence and natural history of dilated cardiomyopathy is incompletely known and the proportion of cases wholly or partially due to alcohol is uncertain. It is therefore impossible to estimate the numerical contribution made to chronic heart muscle disease by alcohol excess or sensitivity. The proportion of heavy drinkers who develop cardiomyopathy is equally obscure, though it has been suggested that 12 units (100 g) of alcohol a day is required for the development of alcoholic heart disease.

Associated Malnutrition

Beri beri heart disease may occur in alcoholics. This is a high output state with rapid heart rate and wide pulse pressure and should not be confused with dilated cardiomyopathy. It usually responds to thiamine. Evidence of thiamine deficiency should be sought in any alcoholic patient with cardiomyopathy and adequate thiamine supplementation given. However, this condition is rarely seen in the United Kingdom.

Toxic effects due to additives

'Beer drinker's cardiomyopathy', a completely separate and now historic disorder, was caused by the addition of cobalt to beer to stabilize the 'head'. Outbreaks of heart failure among heavy beer drinkers were described in the 1960s in Canada.[9] Not all drinkers were affected and susceptibility was associated with malnutrition in heavy labourers who took most of their daily calories as beer. Their health deteriorated rapidly and widespread destruction of heart muscle cells was a feature on microscopy.

Lead in 'moonshine' (illicitly distilled alcohol) has also been implicated in causing cardiomyopathy.

Coronary Heart Disease

A reciprocal relationship between alcohol intake and coronary heart disease has been offered in explanation for the rather low incidence of coronary deaths in the wine-drinking French who have a high death rate from cirrhosis. The protective effect of alcohol is said to be confined to wine but similar benefits have been attributed to garlic.

Recent scientific studies also report that a negative association or even a preventive role exists between moderate alcohol intake and coronary heart disease. A J-shaped curve can be constructed showing a lower incidence of cardiovascular deaths in those who take some alcohol compared with those who either take none or take it to excess. The best information comes from the Whitehall Civil Service Study in which over 18,000 men were observed over ten years.[10] The mortality rate in men drinking moderately was lower than in either non-drinkers or in drinkers who imbibed more than 4 units (32 g) of alcohol a day. Cardiovascular mortality was greater in non-drinkers, and non-cardiovascular mortality was higher in heavy drinkers. This apparent preventive effect of moderate drinking may be spurious because total abstainers may be a special group at higher risk for other reasons.

References

1. Gvozdják, A., Bada, V., Krutý, F., Nederland, T.R., and Gvozdják, J. (1973) Effect of Ethanol on the Metabolism of the Myocardium and its Relationship to Development of Alcoholic Cardiomyopathy. *Cardiology* 58: 290–97.
2. Regan, T.J. and Haider, B. (1981) Ethanol Abuse and Heart Disease. *Circulation* 64: Suppl. III, 14–19.
3. Greenspan, A.J. and Schaal, S.F. (1983) The Holiday Heart. Electrophysiologic Studies of Alcohol Effects in Alcoholics. *Annals of Internal Medicine* 98: 135–39.
4. Schwartz, L., Semple, K.A., and Wigle, E.D. (1975) Severe Alcoholic Cardiomyopathy Reversed with Abstention from Alcohol. *American Journal of Cardiology* 36: 963–66.
5. Rubin, E. (1979) Alcoholic Myopathy in Heart and Skeletal Muscle. *New England Journal of Medicine* 28–33.
6. Brigden, W. and Robinson, J. (1964) Alcoholic Heart Disease. *British Medical Journal* 2: 1283–289.
7. World Health Organisation (1984) *Expert Committee on Cardiomyopathies.* Technical Report Series 697. Geneva: WHO.
8. Demakis, J.G., Proskey, A., Rahimtoola, S.H., Jamil, M., Sutton, G.C., Rosen, K.M., Gunnar, R.M., and Tobin, J.R. (1974) The Natural Course of Alcoholic Cardiomyopathy. *Annals of Internal Medicine* 80: 293–97.
9. Morin, Y. and Daniel, P. (1967) Quebec Beer Drinkers Cardiomyopathy. *Canadian Medical Association Journal* 97: 926–28.
10. Marmot, M.G., Rose, G., Shirley, M.J., and Thomas, B. (1981) Alcohol and Mortality: a J-shaped curve. *Lancet* 1: 580–82.

8

BLOOD PRESSURE

Summary

High alcohol intake is an important and common cause of raised blood pressure. All hypertensive patients should be screened for alcohol excess because, with abstinence, blood pressure settles.

The association between high alcohol intake and raised blood pressure was not generally recognized until the late 1970s. Since that time it has become apparent that alcohol excess is the commonest identifiable underlying cause for the elevation of blood pressure in hypertensive patients.

Epidemiological Evidence

The link between alcohol and hypertension was first noted among French soldiers during the First World War.[1] Little further information was published until the 1960s when surveys in India[2] and Los Angeles[3] demonstrated higher blood pressures in all categories of heavy drinkers and alcohol abusers. Since that time practically every large population study has demonstrated a direct relation between blood pressure and reported alcohol intake and biochemical markers of heavy drinking in the serum.[4] This effect has been shown to be independent of age, sex, ethnic origin, body weight, social class, cigarette consumption, and reported salt preference. The largest and most reliable study was published by Klatsky *et al.*[5] Around 10 per cent of abstainers and light drinkers consuming up to 2.5 units (20 g) of alcohol daily (equivalent to 1.25 pints of beer) had raised blood pressures. By contrast more than 20 per cent of people consuming 15 units (120 g) of alcohol daily were hypertensive (*Figure* 7). There may be a J-shaped relationship, so that people who drink no more than 20 g alcohol daily have slightly lower blood pressures than teetotallers. But above this level of intake there is a positive correlation; the higher the intake the higher the pressure.

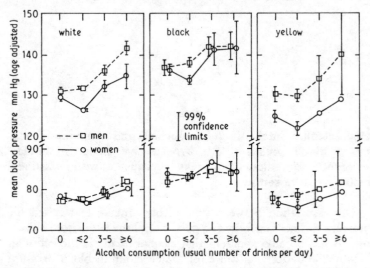

Figure 7 Age adjusted mean systolic and diastolic blood pressure levels according to reported alcohol consumption, by ethnic group and sex. (From Klatsky *et al.* 1977.[5])

Mortality

There is a direct relationship in men between alcohol intake and mortality from all causes.[6] Strokes, which are closely related to hypertension, are three times more common in heavy drinkers than in light drinkers and abstainers. Alcohol-related strokes may occur as a result of raised blood pressure or may be due to constriction of cerebral blood vessels. Around 20 per cent of strokes in young patients are preceded by heavy drinking or alcohol intoxication.[7] Alcohol has also been implicated in subarachnoid haemorrhage (see p. 36).

Coronary heart disease, which is less closely related to hypertension, does not share the same correlation with alcohol intake, as there are fewer heart attacks in moderate drinkers. This protective effect may be due to an effect of alcohol on high-density lipoprotein cholesterol and platelet adhesiveness.[8]

Alcohol Abusers

The prevalence of hypertension is high among people who are heavy drinkers. In a study of 132 alcohol abusers, 46 per cent were found to have raised blood pressure by WHO criteria and 16 per cent had diastolic pressures of 110 mm Hg or more.[9] Thus raised blood pressure of this level is three times more common in heavy drinkers than in the general population.[10]

It is important to note that when hypertensive drinkers stop consuming alcohol, diastolic blood pressure settles by an average of 10 mm Hg, and if they then relapse it rises again.[9]

Hypertensive Patients

Alcohol excess is unduly common among hypertensive patients. Abnormalities of biochemical indices of liver damage and excess alcohol consumption are twice as common as in age and sex matched normotensive controls. Between 30 and 40 per cent of hypertensive patients have raised serum gamma glutamyl transpeptidase (GGT) levels,[11] whereas this abnormality occurs in only about 18 per cent of a control population. When hypertensives who are drinking even moderately stop drinking altogether, their systolic blood pressure falls by an average of 18 mm Hg. If they start to drink again, their blood pressure rises.[12]

Mechanisms

The mechanism(s) of alcohol-related hypertension remain uncertain. It has been shown that in alcohol abusers admitted to hospital, raised blood pressure is related to the occurrence of alcohol withdrawal symptoms rather than to alcohol ingestion itself.[9] The mechanism of this 'alcohol withdrawal hypertension' may differ from the mechanism of the relatively acute rises in blood pressure seen in both hypertensive patients and normal people given an alcohol load of between two and three pints of beer.[13] It may be related to changes in cardiac output, but there is also evidence of constriction of blood vessels in some organs. The rise in blood pressure occurs immediately after ingestion and parallels blood alcohol levels. Various changes in the pressor hormones (catecholamines, renin, angiotensin, and cortisol) have been documented, but these changes occur after the peak rise in blood pressure.

Public Health Considerations

The public health impact of this relatively new clinical observation is great. High blood pressure itself is a very important but treatable risk factor for cardiovascular diseases which in turn cause more premature deaths than all other causes combined. By conservative estimates, about 10 per cent of the population aged 30–60 years have hypertension of a level which should be treated with blood pressure lowering drugs.[10] This represents 2.5 million people in England and Wales. As biochemical evidence of alcohol excess is present in about 30 per cent of hypertensive patients and in about half this number of people with normal blood pressure,[9] it is possible that alcohol accounts for the raised blood pressure in 10–15 per cent of patients with hypertension. This represents between 250,000 and 375,000 individuals. The implications for prevention, particularly of strokes, by reducing alcohol intake are considerable. Total abstinence from alcohol is not necessary, but reduction of a weekly average intake to 'safe' levels (see p. 108) should greatly reduce the prevalence of raised blood pressure and its sequelae.

References

1. Lian, C. (1915) L'Alcoolisme, Cause de Hypertension Artériale. *Bulletin de l'Académie Médicale* (Paris) 74: 525–28.
2. Shah, V.V. (1967) Environmental Factors and Hypertension with Particular Reference to the Prevalence of Hypertension in Alcohol Addicts and Teetotallers. In J. Stamler, R. Stamler, and T. N. Pullman (eds) *The Epidemiology of Hypertension*. New York and London: Grune and Stratton, pp. 204–18.
3. Clark, V.A., Chapman, J.M., and Coulson, A.H. (1967) Effects of Various Factors on Systolic and Diastolic Blood Pressure in the Los Angeles Heart Study. *Journal of Chronic Disease* 20: 571–81.
4. Beevers, D.G. (1977) Alcohol and Hypertension. *Lancet* 2: 114–15.
5. Klatsky, A.L., Friedman, G.D., Sieglaub, A.B., and Gerard, M.J. (1977) Alcohol Consumption and Blood Pressure. Kaiser Permanente Multiphasic Health Examination Data. *New England Journal of Medicine* 296: 1194–200.
6. Kozararevic, D.J., McGee, P., Vojvodic, N., Racic, Z., Dawber, T., Gordon, T., and Zukel, W. (1980) Frequency of Alcohol Consumption and Morbidity and Mortality. The Yugoslavian Cardiovascular Disease Study. *Lancet* 1: 613–16.
7. Hillbom, M. and Kaste, M. (1978) Does Ethanol Intoxication Promote Brain Infarction in Young Adults. *Lancet* 2: 1181–183.
8. Castelli, W.P., Gordon, T., Hjortland, M.C., Kagan, A., Doyle, J.T.,

Hames, C.G., Hulley, S.B. and Zukel, W.J. (1977) Alcohol and Blood Lipids. *Lancet* 2: 153–55.

9. Saunders, J.B., Beevers, D.G., and Paton, A. (1981) Alcohol Induced Hypertension. *Lancet* 2: 653–56.
10. Hawthorne, V.M., Greaves, D.A., and Beevers, D.G. (1974) Blood Pressure in a Scottish Town. *British Medical Journal* 3: 600–03.
11. Potter, J.F., Bannan, L.T., and Beevers, D.G. (1984) Alcohol and Hypertension. *British Journal of Addiction* 79: 49–56.
12. Potter, J.F. and Beevers, D.G. (1984) Pressor Effects of Alcohol in Hypertension. *Lancet* 1: 119–22.
13. Ireland, M.A., Vandongen, R., Davidson, L., Beilin, L.J., and Rouse, I.L. (1984) Acute Effects of Moderate Alcohol Consumption on Blood Pressure and Plasma Catecholamines. *Clinical Science* 66: 643–48.

9

THE CHEST

Summary

Many people who are heavy drinkers or alcohol abusers suffer from breathlessness. This is mainly due to the close association of alcohol intake with cigarette smoking and, in extreme cases, with malnutrition.

The tendency for heavy drinkers also to be heavy smokers probably explains the marked excess of chronic bronchitis and emphysema as well as lung cancer in such people. There is also a higher incidence of tuberculosis.[1] There has been some suggestion that high alcohol intake may hasten the onset of chronic chest disease in smokers.[2] It is uncertain whether the marked excess of cancer deaths in heavy drinkers is due to smoking alone or whether there is some tendency for alcohol itself to promote the development of cancer of the lungs.[3]

Alcohol abusers are frequently malnourished and may also have some depression of their immune system. This has led some observers to postulate the existence of a specific alcohol-induced lung disease, although the evidence for this is poor.[4]

People who frequently become intoxicated tend to fall over and sustain fractures at many sites. The presence of fresh or healed rib fractures on a chest X-ray is often associated with heavy drinking and their presence should alert both clinicians and radiologists to the possibility of alcohol abuse in their patients.[5] People who fall into an alcoholic stupor tend to underbreathe, particularly if they also have rib fractures, and are in danger of developing hypostatic or inhalation pneumonia.[1] There is a possibility that some of the excess incidence of chronic chest disease in heavy drinkers is due to frequent minor episodes of inhalation of vomit. All patients with lobar or bronchopneumonia should be questioned carefully about their alcohol intake.

References

1. Edmonson, H.A. (1980) Pathology of Alcoholism. *American Journal of Clinical Pathology* 74: 728–42.
2. Emirgil, C., Sobol, B.J., Heymann, K., Reed, A., Varble, A., and Waldic, J. (1974) Pulmonary Function in Alcoholics. *American Journal of Medicine* 57: 69–77.
3. Knox, E.G. (1977) Foods and Diseases. *British Journal of the Society for Preventive Medicine* 31: 71–80.
4. Burch, G.E. and de Pasquale, N. (1966) Alcoholic Lung Disease: an Hypothesis. *American Heart Journal* 73: 147–50.
5. Maxwell, J.D., Patel, S.P., Bland, J.M., Lindsell, D.R.M., and Wilson, A.G. (1983) Chest Radiography Compared to Laboratory Markers in the Detection of Alcoholic Liver Disease. *Journal of the Royal College of Physicians* (London) 17: 220–23.

10

ENDOCRINE FUNCTION

Summary

Alcohol misuse affects sexual and reproductive function in men and women; in chronic alcohol abusers the damage can become irreversible. Prolonged alcohol excess causes over-secretion of cortisol from the adrenal glands. It disturbs the control of blood sugar and in diabetic persons taking insulin it can cause severe and prolonged depression of the blood sugar level with irreversible brain damage.

There is a large literature reporting studies of endocrine function in chronic alcohol abusers and in response to acute ingestion of alcohol. The picture is confusing because of the varying degrees of liver damage present in the subjects studied and their nutritional status at the time of study.

Sexual Function

It is said that an alcoholic binge 'provokes the desire but takes away the performance'.[1] Persistent heavy drinking, however, can produce longer lasting sexual changes in both men and women as a result of the direct toxic effects of alcohol on the testes and ovaries and on parts of the brain (the hypothalamus) and the pituitary gland responsible for the release of hormones (gonadotrophins) which stimulate these glands.[2] These effects appear to be independent of the presence of liver disease or nutritional deficiencies. Plasma concentrations of the male sex hormone testosterone are reduced in chronic drinking men, and the concentration of the female sex hormone oestradiol is reduced in women drinkers.

Men complain of loss of libido and potency and may develop shrinking of the testes, a reduction in the size of the penis, diminished or absent sperm formation, loss of sexual hair, and of scrotal wrinkling. In men with alcoholic cirrhosis, additional metabolic disturbances cause hormonal changes which lead to enlargement of the breasts and loss of body hair. The incidence of these changes varies considerably; 40–90 per cent report loss of libido, whilst testicular shrinking is observed in 10–75 per cent.

Women with impaired function of the ovaries become progressively defeminized: they complain of sexual difficulties and of menstrual problems such as irregular periods, heavy menstrual loss, or even complete loss of menstrual bleeding. The ovaries, breasts, and external genitalia shrink, body fat redistributes into a male pattern, and vaginal secretions are lost. The overall incidence of these changes is unknown, although breast atrophy was reported in 75 per cent of women in one series.[3]

Very little is known about the reversibility of the effects of alcohol on sexual and reproductive function: information is only available for men.[4] Impotence will improve in 25–50 per cent of male alcohol abusers who subsequently stop drinking. This improvement is more likely to occur in men whose testes have not shrunk and who retain normal gonadotrophin responses to hormonal stimulation by clomiphene or luteinizing hormone releasing factor. Men with gross testicular shrinking or inadequate hormone responses are unlikely to regain adequate sexual function despite continued abstinence from alcohol. Very little can be done to help them.

Recently it has been shown that reproductive function can be seriously disturbed in men taking even modest amounts of alcohol.[5] Of 67 men attending a male infertility clinic 26 (39 per cent) were thought to have alcohol-related impairment of sperm formation. The majority drank 4–6 units of alcohol (32–48 g, equivalent to 2–3 pints of beer) daily and had not previously abused alcohol. In approximately half the patients semen analysis became normal after three months of abstinence from alcohol and there have been four pregnancies to date. No similar studies are available in women consuming moderate amounts of alcohol.

Adrenal Function

Acute ingestion of alcohol causes release of cortisol from the adrenal glands, mediated by interaction between the pituitary gland and closely associated parts of the brain (the hypothalamus).

The oversecretion of cortisol may produce a clinical syndrome of obesity, increased facial hair, and high blood pressure, closely resembling Cushing's syndrome. It may be difficult to distinguish between true and alcohol-induced Cushing's syndrome. In both plasma and urine cortisol levels are raised, the normal daily rhythm of secretion is lost, and there may be inadequate suppression of the secretion from the pituitary gland of the hormone (ACTH).[6,7] These biochemical abnormalities rapidly revert to normal on withdrawal of alcohol in most cases, but if there is associated mental depression some abnormalities may persist. If drinking is resumed, the abnormalities promptly return.

Thyroid Gland

Alcohol probably has no direct effect on the production of thyroid hormones. However, chronic alcohol abusers may demonstrate a clinical syndrome suggestive of thyroid overactivity with loss of weight, anxiety, palpitations, sweating, and tremor. Biochemical tests should help to distinguish the two, but associated liver disease and/or malnutrition affect the tests in a variety of ways and may cause confusion.[8–9] Serum thyroxine-binding globulin concentration may increase in liver disease with an associated rise in total thyroxine (T_4) and triiodothyronine (T_3) levels; but it may decrease in severely ill patients causing a fall in the concentrations of both hormones. The liver is the major site of the conversion of T_4 to T_3, so that low serum T_3 values are commonly found in drinkers with liver damage. This feature successfully distinguishes them from hyperthyroid patients in whom serum T_3 is almost invariably increased. Chronic alcohol abusers may also exhibit blunting of the control of thyroid gland function by the hypothalamus.[4]

Endocrine Pancreas

Alcohol-Induced Hypoglycaemia

A fall in blood sugar concentration – often profound and occasionally sufficient to cause coma – may follow within 6–36 hours of an alcoholic binge, especially if the alcohol was taken on an empty stomach. Particularly at risk are young children who may finish off the remnants of their parents' drinks on a Sunday morning – the 'Sunday morning syndrome' (see p. 96). Fasting depletes the liver's glycogen stores and alcohol directly inhibits glucose synthesis from amino acids. The hypoglycaemia that may follow is refractory to glucagon. While alcohol seems to have no direct action on insulin release, it augments the plasma insulin increment after glucose ingestion.[10] This usually produces only a transient drop in blood glucose but in some susceptible people may give rise to mild symptoms of hypoglycaemia after consuming a gin and (sugar-containing) tonic, for example.

Diabetes Mellitus

Diabetes does not affect the metabolism of alcohol. It is therefore unnecessary to forbid diabetics to drink alcohol as long as they take into account the energy content (calories) of the beverage (*Table 8*),[11] and, like anyone else, avoid heavy drinking. In insulin-dependent diabetics, the combination of insulin and the inhibition of glucose production by the liver due to excessive alcohol can be lethal. Every year a number of diabetics die or remain severely brain-damaged after heavy drinking despite heroic measures to raise the blood glucose level.[12]

Table 8 *Contents of a typical 'measure' of drink*

beverage	alcohol content (%)	volume (ml)	alcohol (g)	sugar (g)	energy (kcals)
beer, lager	3.5–5.5	280	7.5–12.3	8–15	80–120
'diet lager'	4.0–6.0	280	9.0–13.4	2–10	90–130
wine	10–13	120	9.5	1–3	70–130
dry sherry	18	60	8.5	1.5	65
port	21	45	7.0	5.0	70
spirits	40	24	7.5	0	50
mixers					
regular	0	120	0	10	40
sugar free	0	120	0	0	0

(Reproduced with permission from Wright and Marks, and Rosalki.[11])

Prolonged heavy alcohol ingestion increases the rate of metabolism of drugs such as tolbutamide and chlorpropamide used in the treatment of some diabetics and this may cause deterioration of their diabetic control.

Up to 50 per cent of diabetic patients being treated with chlorpropamide experience an intense facial flush when they drink even a small amount of alcohol.[13,14] It also occurs in non-diabetic volunteers taking chlorpropamide and alcohol. The flush is produced by aldehyde which accumulates in the blood because the activity of the enzyme responsible for its breakdown (acetaldehyde dehydrogenase) is reduced by these drugs.[15] Acetaldehyde also stimulates the release of other agents that cause dilatation of small blood vessels.

Alcohol abuse may sometimes cause clinically overt but relatively mild diabetes, usually accompanied by a sharp increase in the amount of fat in the blood,[16] probably as a result of alcohol-related pancreatitis. Significant glucose intolerance occurs in individuals with alcoholic cirrhosis. It is a complex state in which altered insulin metabolism and a decreased number of hepatic insulin receptors, oversecretion of insulin and of glucagon (which counteracts the effect of insulin on the blood sugar) combine to present a picture of glucose intolerance, a raised fasting blood sugar level, and simultaneously high levels of insulin and glucagon in the blood.[17]

References

1. Shakespeare, W. (1606) In *Macbeth*, Act 2, Scene 3.
2. Morgan, M.Y. (1982) Sex and Alcohol. *British Medical Bulletin* 38: 43–52.
3. Valimaki, M. and Ylikahri, R. (1983) The Effect of Alcohol on Male and Female Sexual Function. *Alcohol and Alcoholism* 18: 313–20.
4. Van Thiel, D.H., Gavalar, J.S., and Sanghvi, A. (1983) Recovery of Sexual Function in Abstinent Alcoholic Men. *Gastroenterology* 84: 677–82.
5. Morgan, M.Y. (1982) The Effects of Moderate Alcohol Consumption on Male Fertility. In M. Langer, L. Chiandussi, J. Chopra, and L. Martini (eds) *The Endocrines and the Liver* (Serono Symposium No. 51). London: Academic Press, pp. 157–58.
6. Smals, A.G., Kloppenborg, P.W., Njo, K.T., Knoben, J.M., and Ruland, C.M. (1976) Alcohol Induced Cushingoid Syndrome. *British Medical Journal* 2: 1298.
7. Rees, L., Besser, G.M., Jeffcoate, W.J., Goldie, D.J., and Marks, V. (1977) Alcohol Induced Pseudo Cushing's Syndrome. *Lancet* i: 726–28.
8. Green, J.R.B., Snitcher, E.J., Mowat, N.A.G., Ekins, R.P., Rees, L.H., and Dawson, A.M. (1977) Thyroid Function and Thyroid Regulation in Euthyroid Man with Chronic Liver Disease. Evidence of Multiple Abnormalities. *Clinical Endocrinology* 7: 453–61.
9. Kallner, G. (1981) Assessment of Thyroid Function in Chronic Alcoholism. *Acta Medica Scandinavica* 209: 93–6.
10. O'Keefe, S.J.D. and Marks, V. (1977) Lunchtime Gin and Tonic – a Cause of Reactive Hypoglycaemia. *Lancet* i: 1286–288.
11. Wright, J. and Marks, V. (1985) The Effects of Alcohol on Carbohydrate

Metabolism. In S. B. Rosalki (ed.) *Clinical Biochemistry of Alcoholism.* Edinburgh: Churchill Livingstone, pp. 135–48.

12. Arky, R.A., Veverbrant, E., and Abramson, E.A. (1968) Irreversible Hypoglycaemia: a Complication of Alcohol and Insulin. *Journal of the American Medical Association* 206: 575–78.

13. Fitzgerald, M.G., Gaddie, R., Malins, J.M., and O'Sullivan, D.J. (1962) Alcohol Sensitivity in Diabetics Receiving Chlorpropamide. *Diabetes* 11: 40–3.

14. Leslie, R.D.G. and Pyke, D.A. (1978) Chlorpropamide-Alcohol Flushing: a Dominantly Inherited Trait Associated with Diabetes. *British Medical Journal* ii: 1519–521.

15. Jerntorp, P., Almer, L-O., and Melander, A. (1981) Is the Chlorpropamide Concentration Critical in CPAF? *Lancet* i: 165–66.

16. Philips, G.B. and Safrit, M.F. (1971) Alcoholic Diabetes: Induction of Glucose Intolerance with Alcohol. *Journal of the American Medical Association* 217: 1513–519.

17. Johnston, D.G. and Alberti, K.G.M.M. (1976) Carbohydrate Metabolism in Liver Disease. *Clinics in Endocrinology and Metabolism* 5: 675–702.

11

OCCUPATION

Summary

Alcohol problems in society at large are also apparent at the workplace. In industry, they take their toll through absenteeism, accidents, poor performance, and poor leadership. Yet the workplace can provide the ideal setting in which those suffering from alcohol problems can be identified and offered help. Employees must be made aware of the dangers of alcohol abuse and employers must translate alcohol policies into practice.

Alcohol and Work

In 1977 the National Council on Alcoholism[1] declared:

'The vast majority of people with a drinking problem are males in full-time employment. The nature of the problem is that it does not conveniently subside on a Monday morning and relapse on a Friday evening: people with drinking problems will bring them to work daily.'

This claim was supported by figures from Edwards's study[2] of clients at Alcohol Information Centres in which he found that 88 per cent of the clients were at times having a drink before going into work; 62 per cent on occasion took a bottle to work; 12 per cent took a bottle to work every day; all but 9 per cent said they would occasionally continue drinking throughout the working day. Moss and Beresford Davies,[3] examining excessive drinking in Cambridgeshire, found that 52 per cent of men drinking to excess developed work problems from drinking, but only 4.2 per cent were unemployable or retired prematurely because of alcohol abuse.

Kenyon[4] has estimated that 75 per cent of problem drinkers are in full-time gainful employment. They are, however, more likely to have accidents at work, take more than average sick leave, produce a poorer than average work performance, and cause more problems to supervisors and managers. Putting a figure on the cost to industry has proved difficult. Holtermann and Burchell[5] put the overall total resource cost of alcohol problems in England and Wales as high as £650 million in 1977 or over £1000 million at 1984 prices. The most recent estimate[6] is that the days lost to industry through alcohol-related problems cost the country £641 million a year.

Absenteeism

Edwards et al.[2] found that 98 per cent of his clients admitted losing an average of 68 days a year from work due to drinking. Sixty-six per cent admitted that they were often late for work and 61 per cent reported absence on Monday mornings. Wilson[7] found that a much higher proportion of heavy drinkers than of light or moderate drinkers reported being off work for more than three days because of illness in the previous three months.

Saad and Madden[8] found an average yearly time loss of 121.7 working days per person in seventy-three alcoholic men in Merseyside, 86.1 days through sickness and 35.6 days through unemployment. By contrast, the average absence because of sickness for employed men in a comparable period was 15.9 days. It is surprising that out of 149 certificated sickness absences there were only five diagnoses of alcohol abuse or delirium tremens. This may be due to a desire by doctors to avoid embarrassing patients or to patients' ability to hide excessive drinking from doctors. It illustrates the difficulties of accurate assessment of the extent of the problem associated with alcohol, the stigma associated with it and its concealment.

Accidents at Work

The Blennerhassett committee[9] demonstrated the relationship between drunken driving and traffic accidents, yet little attention has been paid by the legislature to the effects of drinking at work. In the Robens Report on Health and Safety at Work no mention was made of alcohol as a possible cause of accidents, though certain sections of the 1974 Health and Safety at Work Act can be interpreted to cover aspects of alcohol-related problems in employment.[10]

Various research studies have demonstrated the increased likelihood of accidents at work in heavy drinkers. Eleven per cent of

Edwards's clients admitted that their alcohol consumption had been responsible for an accident at work and 32 per cent thought their drinking might have contributed to one.[2] Davies[11] found that 21 per cent of men interviewed in a shipyard, a brewery, and a manufacturing industry on Clydeside had knowledge of alcohol-related accidents.

Accidents may occur not only to problem drinkers, but also to workers who drink at lunchtime and then operate heavy machinery. It is known that anyone who consumes three pints of beer or its equivalent (6 units) before driving is up to six times more likely to have an accident; the same is presumably true of those drinking and working in a dangerous environment. Wilson[7] found that one in ten men and one in twenty women in full-time employment reported feeling the effects of a hangover while at work or doing their housework.

Alcohol also affects judgement and decision-making so that the obvious accidents on the shop floor may be paralleled by bad leadership and ineffective management through alcohol abuse in the board room or the executive suite. These are largely invisible 'accidents' yet their effect may be more far-reaching than those confined to the shop floor.

Conditions at the Workplace

A major factor in the damage to industry caused by alcohol abuse is the variable approach taken by employers to alcohol consumption by the workforce. At one end of the scale, companies operating North Sea oil rigs ban alcohol completely and send back anyone reporting for duty under the influence of alcohol. At the other end, the distillers have only recently ceased the process of 'dramming' – the provision of up to one gill of strong spirits (4–8 units, depending on local custom) as a daily 'perk' for each worker – though some brewers still accept the argument of their sales representatives that 'if we don't drink it we can't sell it'.

Three factors which Plant[12] has identified may contribute to a tendency to abuse alcohol – availability, social pressures to drink, and separation from normal social or sexual relationships. To these, Murray[13] adds freedom from supervision. Certain high-risk occupations may attract workers who are already heavy drinkers.[12] Employees must recognize and guard against these increased risks. This will be difficult if employers are unwilling to lay down firm guidelines as to what is or is not acceptable drinking among staff. In fact, management may unwittingly encourage drinking through refusal to take a stand. It will also be difficult to warn of the dangers if:

1. it is normal practice for employees to consume alcohol before reporting for work or during rest periods;
2. a bar is provided where alcohol is available at subsidized rates and whose profits are ploughed back into a 'sport and social club';
3. alcohol is provided free of charge for executive management under the guise of a 'hospitality' or 'entertainment' allowance;
4. it is normal for alcohol to be available and consumed at in-house meetings and when entertaining visiting clients or customers.

Physical factors

Persons doing heavy physical work, especially those exposed to heat, may suffer dehydration and attempt to relieve the associated thirst with alcohol. Dust and fumes may also contribute. Occupations that are particularly affected are iron and steel workers, miners, and dockers.[14]

Chemical factors

Cerebral depressants potentiate the effects of alcohol, leading to decreased levels of awareness in individuals exposed to solvents (e.g. trichlorethylene, xylene, and toluene) and styrene. A particular interaction between trichlorethylene and alcohol produces drunkenness after consumption of small amounts of alcohol, and skin blotches due to vasodilatation – 'degreaser's flush'.[15] Some substances, such as calcium cyanamide, may affect alcohol metabolism and cause the appearance of toxic metabolites. Thiurams used in the manufacture of synthetic rubber and fungicides may cause an Antabuse reaction with alcohol because they inhibit the metabolism of alcohol[16] (see Appendix 3).

Medication

Many workers, for example those with high blood pressure or diabetes, can only stay in regular and effective employment with the aid of short-term or maintenance drug therapy. Those who consume alcohol in addition may risk their health and work performance because of the interaction of alcohol and drugs (see Appendix 3).

Policies on Alcohol at Work

Until comparatively recently problem drinking at work has been dealt with either by collusion or by dismissal.[17] In the last few years an increasing number of employers have adopted policies aimed at the early identification, treatment, and rehabilitation of employees who abuse alcohol. These are based on identification by absenteeism, poor work performance, and unacceptable behaviour; counselling by heads of departments or representatives of welfare or personnel staff; and enrolment in recovery programmes either within the company or in outside specialist organizations.

Provision is made for employees who believe they have an alcohol problem to consult occupational health or welfare services. While undergoing a recovery programme, an employee is regarded as being on sick leave; help is given in the strictest confidence and job security is guaranteed. In the final resort, such a referral may be offered as an alternative to dismissal. About 75 per cent of people defined as having an alcohol problem are in gainful employment. Unfortunately there is relatively little information on which to judge the success of occupational alcohol policies, though success has been claimed in rehabilitating a majority of those identified and treated. A 'success rate' of up to 70 per cent compares favourably with those achieved in alcohol treatment elsewhere.[18]

Measured against other criteria, alcohol policies appear to be less successful. Only a small proportion of those with alcohol problems are identified; and most schemes are unable to identify alcohol abuse at an early enough stage. These difficulties may be explained by a number of factors. First, there may be reluctance among managers to confront alcohol misuse for fear that their own drinking may be called into question. Second, factors within the workplace which encourage drinking on or before duty, tend to render problem drinking less socially visible. Third, those involved in a staff welfare and occupational health service complain that managers are often ineffective because they avoid the issue until the situation has deteriorated beyond retrieval. But managers are often given little instruction in how to cope with alcohol abuse; when they have undergone training they are likely to be more effective.[18] Finally, if employees are to be encouraged to refer themselves for help, they must be made aware that a policy exists and must be informed of the early signs of an alcohol problem.

Education and Training

Such limited evidence as is available[19] shows a surprising ignorance among the workforce concerning the nature and effects of alcohol; this may represent a lack of knowledge in the country generally.[20] As most of the adult population of working age is still in full or part-time employment, the workplace provides an ideal context in which health education on alcohol can be undertaken. It may be more effective to provide it in the wider context of information about smoking, diet and heart disease, exercise, and so on. Where an employer has implemented an alcohol policy it is important that its existence and content is made known to everyone.

Education should include:

1. information on the alcohol content of different drinks;
2. information on the effect of alcohol on the body, the time taken to metabolize it, the legal limit for driving, and so on;
3. the dangers of excess alcohol consumption, acute and chronic, at home as well as at work;
4. a sensible limit for alcohol consumption on a daily/weekly basis;
5. a chart to help employees judge whether they are drinking to excess;
6. tips on how they can reduce consumption;
7. the names of people and organizations, at the workplace or elsewhere, from whom they can obtain help.

Once the educational content has been decided upon, appropriate methods of delivery should include:

1. booklets/leaflets distributed to each member of staff;
2. posters put up where employees are sure to see them;
3. films of the problems attendant on alcohol abuse;
4. health education exhibitions.

Both managers and shop stewards will face difficulties in implementing an alcohol policy unless guidance is provided. Topics that might be considered in training are:

1. alcohol, the individual, and society;
2. alcohol and work;
3. reducing the problem;

4. identifying the problem drinker;
5. interviewing the problem drinker;
6. guidance and help.

References

1. Braine, B. (1977) *Report of the Working Party on Alcohol and Work.* London: National Council on Alcoholism.
2. Edwards, G., Kelloy-Fisher, M., Hawker, A., and Hensaman, C. (1967) Clients of Alcoholism Information Centres. *British Medical Journal* 4: 346–49.
3. Moss, M.C. and Beresford Davies, E. (1967) *A Survey of Alcoholism in an English County.* London: Geigy (UK).
4. Kenyon, W.M. (1979) *Company Policies and Programmes.* Liverpool: Merseyside, Lancashire and Cheshire Council on Alcoholism, 16th Annual Report 1979.
5. Holtermann, S. and Burchell, A. (1981) *Government Economic Service Working Paper.* No. 37. London: DHSS.
6. Maynard, A. (1985) Alcohol Use: Costs and Benefits. *Alcohol Concern* 1: 11–12.
7. Wilson, R. (1980) *Drinking Patterns in England and Wales.* London: HMSO.
8. Saad, E.S.M. and Madden, J.S. (1976) Certificated Incapacity and Unemployment in Alcoholics. *British Journal of Psychiatry* 128: 340–45.
9. Department of the Environment (1976) *Departmental Committee Report: Drinking and Driving.* London: HMSO.
10. Scottish Council on Alcoholism (1981) *Alcohol and Employment. A Report of the Working Party on Alcohol in Employment.* Glasgow.
11. Davies, J.B. (1981) Drinking and Alcohol-Related Problems in Five Industries. In B. D. Hore and M. A. Plant (eds) *Alcohol Problems in Employment.* London: Croom Helm, pp. 38–60.
12. Plant, M.A. (1977) Occupational Factors in Alcoholism. In M. Grant and W. H. Kenyon (eds) *Alcoholism and Industry.* Liverpool: Merseyside Alcohol Education Centre, pp. 28–33.
13. Murray, R.M. (1975) Alcoholism and Employment. *Journal of Alcoholism* 10: 23–6.
14. Godard, J. (1983) Alcoholism. In *ILO Encyclopaedia of Occupational Health and Safety,* 3rd edn. Geneva: International Labour Organisation.
15. David, A. (1983) Trichloroethylene. In *ILO Encyclopaedia of Occupational Health and Safety,* 3rd edn. Geneva: International Labour Organisation.
16. Malten, K.E. (1983) Tetramethyl Thiuram Disulphide. In *ILO Encyclopaedia of Occupational Health and Safety,* 3rd edn. Geneva: International Labour Organisation.
17. Health and Safety Executive (1981) *The Problem Drinker at Work. HSE Occasional Paper Series OP1.* London: HMSO.
18. Hyman, J. and Beaumont, P.B. (forthcoming) *Problem Drinking at Work: Identifying the Problem.* Glasgow: Department of Social and Economic Research, University of Glasgow.

19. Cyster, R. and McEwen, J. (1984) Alcohol Education at the Workplace. Paper delivered at 21st International Congress on Occupational Health, Dublin.
20. WHICH? (1984) *Alcohol and Your Health*. London: Consumer Association.

12

INJURIES

Summary

Alcohol abuse is the single most important factor contributing to bodily damage and adds considerably to the severity of the injuries that may be sustained. The role played by alcohol in deaths due to motor vehicle accidents is well known; excessive levels of alcohol are found in half of the fatalities. It is also a major contributor to pedestrian accidents, to falls, attempted suicides, assaults, and murder. Although there have been improvements over the last two decades in reducing casualties from drinking and driving, tighter legislative controls together with greater public awareness of the problem could produce a dramatic reduction in the number of road accidents.

Injuries are the largest health problem in the United Kingdom between the ages of one and forty years, and account for more deaths during adolescence than all other causes.

Alcohol intoxication is a common finding among patients attending accident and emergency departments. For example, at the Royal Infirmary, Edinburgh, 32 per cent of patients had blood alcohol concentrations above 80 mg/100 ml.[1] Alcohol increases the risk of an accident by reducing coordination of movement, slowing reaction time, blurring vision, decreasing awareness, impairing ability to judge speed and distances, and giving a false sense of confidence in performing skilled tasks.

Road Traffic Accidents

The most common form of alcohol-related trauma is road traffic accident. As early as 1904 it was reported in the USA: 'In 19 out of 25 fatal accidents occurring to automobile wagons . . . drivers had used spirits within an hour or more of the disaster'.[2]

Three distinct groups – problem drinkers, teenagers, and heavy social drinkers – make up the majority of persons in alcohol-related traffic accidents. In this context, problem drinkers are those who have had more than one arrest for offences involving alcohol and who are known to have a history of troubled relationships with employers and families. They make up about two-thirds of those arrested for alcohol-impaired driving.[3] Teenagers tend to have more accidents than adults when the blood alcohol concentration is below 80 mg/100 ml, confirming that inexperience in drinking and inexperience in driving are a bad combination.

At the Burns Unit of the Birmingham Accident Hospital the overall incidence of pre-accident drinking was 18 per cent compared with an expected figure of 2 per cent;[4] 40 per cent of the victims of road traffic accidents had been drinking. Over 9600 drivers involved in accidents causing injuries had positive roadside screening tests for raised blood alcohol. At least one driver had a positive screening test in 45 per cent of accidents in which a driver or passenger was seriously injured.[5]

The risk of having an accident after drinking depends on the blood alcohol concentration and the driver's own susceptibility to its effects[6] (*Figure 8*). There are marked regional differences in the frequency of alcohol-associated road traffic accidents. *Table 9* presents the proportion of persons killed on the roads in Great Britain in 1983–84 who had blood alcohol levels in excess of 80 mg/100 ml and 150 mg/100 ml.[7] The differences between pedestrians and pedal cyclists are especially noticeable.

Warren *et al.*[8] confirmed previous observations that alcohol-related crashes tend to cluster at the top of the severity scale both in

Table 9 *Persons aged 16 and over killed in Britain within twelve hours of a road traffic accident according to blood alcohol level 1983–84*

	drivers	riders	passengers	pedestrians	pedal cyclists
% in excess of 80 mg/100 ml	30	25	32	29	7
% in excess of 150 mg/100 ml	19	17	16	21	4
no. in sample	1454	994	808	1182	186

(*Source*: Department of Transport (1984) *Road Accidents in Great Britain*. London: HMSO.[7])

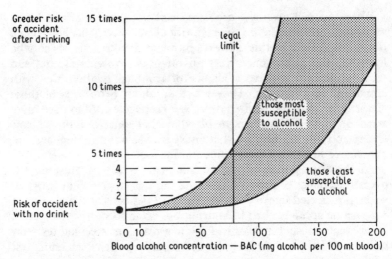

Figure 8 Blood alcohol levels and the risk of accidents.[6]

terms of personal injury and property damage. The common situation is that the intoxicated driver brakes too late and in an uncontrolled way. The cost of alcohol-related road traffic accidents is considerable: McDonnell and Maynard[9] have estimated a figure of the order of £178 million a year, of which £89 million is for material damage.

Pedestrians are clearly not blameless. Clayton *et al.*[10] compared the distribution of the blood alcohol concentrations of adult pedestrian fatalities with matched control samples from uninvolved pedestrians. They give a relative risk of having a fatal accident of 4.6 for pedestrians with a blood alcohol concentration greater than 80 mg/100 ml; in Belfast[11] the figure was 3.6. People in accidents associated with drinking had more severe injuries.

Honkanen and Visuri[12] have shown that head injuries were more likely to be associated with alcohol (47 per cent) than were arm injuries (25 per cent); 39 per cent of tibial and ankle fractures were also associated with alcohol. Head and legs are clearly at risk in drunken persons, so that not only driving but even walking while intoxicated increases the risk of an accident. Fractured ribs following falls due to intoxication are also a common injury.

Development of Legal Controls for Drinking and Driving

The dangers arising from riders and drivers being in charge of their vehicles while under the influence of drink have long been recognized and various laws have been enacted to make it an offence (e.g. the Licensing Act 1872). Similar safeguards were incorporated in the Road Traffic Acts of the present century but it became increasingly clear that although alcohol was a contributory factor in many accidents, the drivers concerned frequently escaped prosecution because the only evidence of their impairment was dubious or lacking, and only those cases in which the offence was obvious were prosecuted.

No specific blood alcohol level was prescribed at which impairment was assumed to begin. Therefore it was often difficult to obtain sufficiently firm evidence to secure a conviction and drivers with high concentrations of alcohol were often acquitted. For this reason fewer than one per cent of drivers involved in injury accidents were reported by the police to have contributed to the accidents because of drink. The fact that the problem was much more serious than the official figures suggested became well known to the police and to the medical profession.

An extensive survey made in 1962–63 in Grand Rapids, in the USA, showed that the risk of accident was significantly higher for drivers with blood alcohol concentrations above 80 mg/100 ml, the risk rapidly rising for levels exceeding 100 mg/100 ml.[13] The increase in risk from high alcohol levels is greater for young and elderly drivers than for middle-aged drivers; it is also greater at low alcohol levels for those who rarely or never drink alcohol than for those who drink regularly.

On 9 October 1967 the provisions of a new Road Safety Act came into effect. Part I prescribed a maximum permissible level of 80 mg of alcohol/100 ml of blood and laid down the circumstances in which drivers could be required to provide blood or urine samples for test. A roadside screening by breath test, using an officially approved 'breathalyzer' (the 'Alcotest'), was also introduced to show whether reasonable grounds existed for the police to require the full analysis. The driver could only be tested by breathalyzer by a police constable in uniform, who must have had reason to suspect that the driver had been drinking or had been involved in an accident or had committed a moving traffic offence.

The penalty for driving with more than the legal limit of alcohol in the blood was a compulsory disqualification from driving for at least twelve months and a fine of up to £100 or up to four months imprisonment. The last mentioned penalty was rarely used and the main deterrent was almost certainly disqualification.

There were immediate and substantiated reductions in the absolute numbers of road casualties.[14] In October, November, and December of 1967 total road casualties in Great Britain were 12 per cent, 13 per cent, and 21 per cent fewer than in the corresponding months of 1966. During the twelve months which followed, road fatalities fell by 15 per cent and total casualties by 11 per cent. Of the estimated 12,300 fatal and serious casualties avoided in the period, some 8800 lives were saved during the peak hours for drink-related accidents (10 pm to 4 am).

Two other related factors are likely to have contributed to the reduction in casualties:

1. the widespread publicity and discussion about road safety in the Press, radio, and television;
2. a massive official publicity campaign carried out in the autumn of 1967 to inform the public of the new legal requirements and the reasons for them.

At least two-thirds of the overall reductions were attributed directly to the Act and the surrounding publicity.[14] It was drinking behaviour rather than driving behaviour or total alcohol intake that was affected by the legislation because during this period national consumption of alcohol and motor traffic continued to increase.

Table 10 *Motor vehicle riders and drivers killed in England and Wales within twelve hours of an accident. (Data supplied by coroners.)*

	sample size	percentage with blood alcohol exceeding (mg per 100 ml)					
		9	50	80	100	150	200
before Road Safety Act:							
Dec. 1966–Sept. 1967	544	37	29	29	22	13	6
after Road Safety Act:							
Dec. 1967–Sept. 1968	389	26	17	15	14	10	4
Dec. 1968–Sept. 1969	454	29	22	19	17	11	5
Dec. 1969–Sept. 1970	449	29	23	20	16	12	6

Table 10 shows the result of a study carried out by the Transport and Road Research Laboratory on the blood alcohol content of motor vehicle riders and drivers who died within twelve hours of an accident. Reports from coroners in England and Wales revealed important and highly statistically significant reductions in the

proportion of drivers with raised blood alcohol levels. Sadly however, by 1972 the effect of the legislation had largely worn off. Alcohol-related accidents increased to levels higher than those experienced prior to 1967.

As a consequence of the increasing number of accidents involving alcohol and the growing exploitation of legal loopholes in the legislation, a Government Committee of Enquiry into Drinking and Driving was set up in 1974. Known as the Blennerhassett Committee after its Chairman, it reported in 1976. However, other than minor alterations to penalties, it was not until the 1981 Road Traffic Act that the legislation was further improved.

Provision has now been made for the use of electronic breath sampling equipment, and the simplified prosecution process closes many loopholes. The number of acquittals resulting from failure to observe technical requirements of the law will therefore be reduced. However the Blennerhasset Committee's recommendation concerning random breath testing has yet to reach the statute book.

There seems little doubt today that a greater awareness of the dangers which result from drinking and driving, together with tighter legislation controls and a wider understanding of alcohol-related problems could produce a dramatic reduction in the number of accidents on roads with a consequent saving in life and limb.

Industrial Accidents

This area is less well documented, especially in the United Kingdom. In the United States as many as one-third of industrial accidents can be related to alcohol abuse at the workplace.[15] Observer and Maxwell[16] showed that among 10,000 subjects the accident rate of a group who abused alcohol was three times that of a control group. Among 20,000 French industrial workers, 7 per cent of accidents were caused by alcohol, and when accidents serious enough to stop work were considered, the rate rose to 15 per cent.[17] Legarde and Hudson[18] found that alcohol was involved in half of twenty fatalities following accidents with farm machinery.

Aviation Accidents

Alcohol appears to be less involved in fatal aircraft accidents, particularly military,[19] but, as with road accidents, the continuing problem lies with the excessive drinker.[20] This was confirmed by Lacefield et al.[21] in a study of 1345 fatal general aviation accidents from 1968–74 in the USA.

Domestic Accidents

Home accidents put a heavy burden on the National Health Service: the Royal Society for the Prevention of Accidents (ROSPA) estimated that in 1984–85 they cost £160 million. Alcohol is believed to be an important contributory factor in about one-third of all domestic accidents.[22] The Department of Trade's Consumer Safety Unit[23] published information obtained from Coroner's files about personal factors in domestic accidents. In 1977, 3 per cent of fatal accidents in the home were alcohol-related in those aged 65 and over; for those aged 15–64 alcohol was implicated in 26 per cent, the commonest types being falls and overdoses. Alcohol was implicated in 39 per cent of deaths from fires; other studies have found even higher proportions, for example, 54 per cent in Scotland[24] and 80 per cent in Strathclyde.[25]

Drowning

Alcohol was a factor in 15 per cent of drownings in the United Kingdom in 1974–75.[26] These deaths comprised drunken men falling in from waterside paths on their way home and seamen falling into harbours when returning to their ships. There was also a group of young men who had gone swimming for fun after drinking heavily. In 1980, 809 deaths by drowning were reported in England and Wales;[26] alcohol was reported as a major contributing factor in 26 per cent of those aged 15–64. The 'sudden drowning syndrome' describes a fatal combination of cold water, alcohol, and non-swimming sportsmen: such deaths are not uncommon in South Africa and Australia.

Suicide and Homicide

The suicide rate among alcohol abusers is fifty-eight times that of the general population, and 30 per cent of persons who take their own lives are excessive drinkers. In Scotland, alcohol is involved in 60 per cent of attempted suicides.[27] Under the influence of alcohol those predisposed to suicide overcome their inhibitions and so become more impulsive and more damaging than they would be when sober: this is evident in the destructiveness of the methods used when intoxicated.[28]

Some alcohol abusers who demonstrate extrovert aggressive behaviour can be extremely dangerous. In the West of Scotland, 50 per cent of homicides involved alcohol, with nearly 50 per cent of the victims also being intoxicated.[29] In ninety-two homicides in Helsinki, alcohol was present in 79 per cent of the victims or perpetrators. In most cases, both were under the influence of alcohol and the levels were high, averaging over 200 mg/100 ml.[30] Investigations of criminal homicide show that aggressive behaviour is just as often initiated by the victim as the perpetrator.[31] Murderers are rarely alcohol abusers and homicide is associated with intoxication rather than with chronic abuse. The triad of familiarity, weapons, and alcohol is the common ingredient of serious assaults which are normally sudden impulsive acts. Alcohol is related to violent crime far more than any other drug.

References

1. Holt, S., Stewart, I.C., Dixon, J.M.J., Elton, R.A., Taylor, T.V., and Little, K. (1980) Alcohol and the Emergency Service Patient. *British Medical Journal* 281: 638–40.
2. Secretary to the Department of Transportation (1968) *Alcohol and Highway Safety*. Washington DC: US Government Printing Office.
3. Maull, K.I. (1982) Alcohol Abuse: its Implications in Trauma Care. *Southern Medical Journal* 75: 794–98.
4. White, A.C. (1980) Drinking and Accidents. A Study of Pre-Accident Drinking and Total Alcohol Consumption in a Sample of Accident Hospital Patients. In J. S. Madden, R. Walker and W. H. Kenyan (eds) *Aspects of Alcohol and Drug Dependence*. London: Pitman Medical.
5. Sabey, B.E. (1978) *A Review of Drinking and Drug-Taking in Road Accidents in Great Britain*. Suppl. Report 41. Crowthorne, Berks: Transport and Road Research Laboratory.
6. Transport and Road Research Laboratory (1983) *The Facts about Drinking and Driving*. Crowthorne, Berks: Transport and Road Research Laboratory.
7. Department of Transport (1984) *Road Accidents in Great Britain*. London: HMSO.
8. Warren, R.A., Simpson, H.M., Buhlman, M.A. *et al.* (1981) Relationship of Driver Blood Alcohol to Injury Severity. 25th Proceedings of the American Association of Automotive Medicine, 1–3 October, San Francisco.
9. McDonnell, R. and Maynard, A. (1985) The Costs of Alcohol Misuse. *British Journal of Addiction* 80: 27–35.
10. Clayton, A.B., Booth, A.C., and McCarthy, P.E. (1977) *A Controlled Study of the Role of Alcohol in Fatal Adult Pedestrian Accidents*. *Suppl. Report 332*. Crowthorne, Berks: Transport and Road Research Laboratory.
11. Irwin, S.T., Patterson, C.C., and Rutherford, W.H. (1983) Association Between Alcohol Consumption and Adult Pedestrians who Sustain

Injuries in Road Traffic Accidents. *British Medical Journal* 286: 522.
12. Honkanen, R. and Visuri, T. (1976) Blood Alcohol Levels in a Series of Injured Patients with Special Reference to Accident and Type of Injury. *Annales Chirurgica Gynaecologica* 65: 287–94.
13. Borkenstein, R.F. (1964) *The Role of the Drinking Driver in Traffic Accidents*. Indiana, Ill.: Indiana University.
14. Newby, R.F. (1971) Casualty Reductions in Great Britain Following the Road Safety Act 1967. Paper presented at OECD International Symposium 1971. London: BMA House.
15. Pell, S. and D'Alonzo, C.A. (1970) Sickness Absenteeism of Alcoholics. *Journal of Occupational Medicine* 6: 198–210.
16. Observer, A. and Maxwell, M.A. (1959) A Study of Absenteeism. Accidents and Sickness Payments in Problem Drinkers in One Industry. *Quarterly Journal of Studies in Alcoholism*. 20: 302–12.
17. Metz, B. and Marcoux, F. (1960) Alcoolization et Accidents du Travail. *Revue de L'Alcool* 6: 3–6.
18. Legarde, J.C. and Hudson, P. (1975) Accidental Deaths with Farm Machinery. *Carolina Forensic Bulletin* 22: 1–4.
19. Davis, G.L. (1968) Alcohol and Military Aviation Fatalities. *Clinical Aviation and Aerospace Medicine* 39: 869–72.
20. Ryan, L.C. and Mohler, S.R. (1972) Intoxicating Liquor and the General Aviation Pilot in 1971. *Clinical Aviation and Aerospace Medicine* 43: 1024–026.
21. Lacefield, D.J., Roberts, P.A., and Blossom, S.W. (1975) Toxicology Findings in Fatal Civilian Aviation Accidents. *Aviation, Space and Environmental Medicine* 46: 1030–034.
22. Taylor, D. (1981) *Alcohol: Reducing the Harm*. London: Office of Health Economics.
23. Department of Trade (1980) *Personal Factors in Domestic Accidents*. London: Consumer Safety Unit.
24. Scottish Council on Alcoholism (1977) *Annual Report*. Edinburgh: SCA.
25. Strathclyde Regional Council (1981) *Firemasters' Report*. Glasgow: SRC.
26. Home Office (1981) *Statistics of Drownings: England and Wales, Statistical Bulletin 17/18, 28 July*. London: HMSO.
27. Platt, S. (1983) Parasuicide. Paper presented at the First Scottish School in Drug Problems. Edinburgh: Heriot-Watt University.
28. Beck, A.T., Weissman, A., and Kovaks, M. (1976) Alcoholism, Hopelessness and Suicidal Behaviour. *Journal of the Study of Alcoholism* 37: 66–77.
29. Gilles, H. (1976) Homicide in the West of Scotland. *British Journal of Psychiatry* 128: 105–08.
30. Hagnell, O., Nyman, E., and Tunvirg, K. (1973) Dangerous Alcoholics. *Scandinavian Journal of Social Medicine* 3: 125–31.
31. Virkkunen, M. (1974) Alcohol as a Factor Perpetrating Aggression and Conflict Behaviour Leading to Homicide. *British Journal of Addiction* 69: 149–54.

13

CHILDREN, ADOLESCENTS, AND THE FAMILY

Summary

Ingestion of alcohol by pregnant women can permanently damage the fetus, leading to abnormal facial features, abnormal growth, and mental retardation. Infants accidentally poisoning themselves and schoolchildren experimenting with alcohol are not infrequently admitted to hospital and occasionally are left permanently brain-damaged as a result of long-lasting, very low blood sugar levels, low body temperature, or lack of oxygen, all induced by alcohol. As expected, children of parents who abuse alcohol experience more than their fair share of problems.

The Unborn Child

Alcohol, like any other drug or chemical taken by the pregnant woman, may:

1. damage the genetic material of the infant in the early phases of development;
2. interfere with organ formation in the embryo stage (16–24 days old) causing structural abnormalities;
3. restrict development of the rapidly growing tissues during the fetal stage (73–280 days old), especially the brain.

The separate effects on the embryo and the fetus are difficult to disentangle; for convenience we have used the labels 'fetal alcohol syndrome' or 'fetal alcohol effects' for both.

Influence on the Genetic Material of the Sperm Cell or Ovum

Several studies on the white blood cells of heavy drinkers have shown that the chromosomes which hold the genetic material may be altered.[1] Furthermore, blood alcohol levels in animals within the range of the heavy human drinker interfere with the genetic make-up of as much as 20 per cent of the sex cells (gametes).[2] It remains to be seen if these findings are relevant to humans.

Most human fetuses with abnormal chromosomes abort spontaneously. It is known that women who drink heavily have about a two-fold increase in risk of spontaneous abortion.[3] The risk of recurrent abortions is even higher. Women taking 1–2 units (8–16 g) of alcohol daily in the first three months of pregnancy appear twice as likely as non-drinkers to have a spontaneous abortion in the second trimester. It remains to be seen whether alcohol is in fact the cause of this increase in abortion rate or merely an associated factor.

Stillbirths and Neonatal Mortality

There is no conclusive evidence that drinking in pregnancy influences the rate of stillbirth. Early reports on small numbers suggested increased neonatal mortality rates in association with alcohol abuse but subsequent large epidemiological enquiries have not revealed such an association.[3]

The Newborn Child

Fetal Alcohol Syndrome

Heavy alcohol consumption in pregnancy, that is more than 10 units (80 g) a day, is associated with the fetal alcohol syndrome.[4] Four major features of the syndrome have been established: intrauterine growth retardation, typical facial features, neuro-developmental abnormalities, and a variety of congenital malformations. The Fetal Alcohol Study Group of the Research Society on Alcoholism defined criteria for diagnosis of the condition.[5]

Growth retardation is symmetrical, and affects the baby's head size. The average birth weight of 2179 g (4 lb 13 oz) is well below the predicted mean for the normal population, that is 3180 g (7 lbs 1 oz). This pattern suggests early intrauterine influences rather than a late 'malnutrition' mechanism, a concept supported by the lack of 'catch-up' in later growth, even when the children are raised in an ideal environment.[6]

The *facial features* of fetal alcohol syndrome are said to be distinctive, but may not always be recognized. The eyes may be small with a short fissure between the lids and prominent folds at the corners. The mid-face is poorly formed, with a short upturned nose with a flattened nasal bridge and prominent nostrils. The vertical groove running from the base of the nose to the upper lip is often absent or poorly formed and the upper lip is thin. The ears may be large, low set, and posteriorly rotated. Similar features have been induced in fetal animals by maternal alcohol exposure.

Mental handicap is the most important effect. The mean IQ of the children concerned is about 70 (mild mental handicap level) although the range is wide. Children with the most severe dysmorphic features and growth retardation usually show the most severe degrees of development delay.[7] Follow-up studies suggest that the deficits remain relatively stable. Such children have small heads, presumably reflecting poor brain growth. Cranial circumference, however, is often in proportion to their general growth deficiency, so that they are not 'microcephalic' in the true sense of that term. Post-mortem studies have shown that brain formation is disorganized, with disturbances of neuronal migration and integration.[8] A variety of neurological problems are commonly found in these children, including epilepsy, unsteadiness, spasticity, or poor muscle tone, and impairment of fine movements. Hyperactive behaviour has also been reported: whether this is a direct effect of prenatal alcohol exposure, the postnatal environment, or other as yet unknown factors, remains to be seen.

Various congenital abnormalities have been reported in association with the fetal alcohol syndrome. Heart defects have been detected in about half the children: the majority of these are proven or presumptive septal defects.[6] Renal and urogenital abnormalities are reported in 12 per cent. Skeletal defects are common; the majority are minor and include poorly formed nails, shortened fingers (usually the fifth), fusion of the bones in the arm and of the fingers or toes.[9] Abnormal crease patterns in the palms of the hands are also found.

Fetal Alcohol Effects

There seems no doubt that heavy alcohol drinking in pregnant women is related to the production of the fetal alcohol syndrome. 'Heavy' is generally taken as at least 6 units (48 g) of alcohol daily and many women with affected children drank much more than this. It is also evident that many women who regularly consume large quantities of alcohol may produce seemingly unaffected children.[3]

Why some mothers produce affected children and others, drinking at the same level, do not, is unknown. In addition some children exhibit only some of the clinical features associated with the fetal alcohol syndrome. These infants are considered to exhibit fetal alcohol effects. In general, such children tend to be growth retarded, have a variety of minor and some major congenital abnormalities, have learning difficulties and behaviour problems, but lack the facial characteristics of the full-blown syndrome.[9]

Incidence of the Fetal Alcohol Syndrome and Fetal Alcohol Effects

An assessment of the overall incidence of the syndrome is not easy. Much depends on the background characteristics of the population under study. There is obvious danger in extrapolating relatively high incidence figures from small atypical communities to produce an artificially inflated frequency for a whole country. The incidence of both is likely to be directly related to the background drinking habits of the population under study. In addition, socioeconomic and/or genetic factors specific to that population may have a strong bearing on the final incidence figures. Estimates of their overall incidence for a whole country, or even region, should therefore be interpreted with caution. With this proviso, published data would suggest that the worldwide incidence of this syndrome appears to be 1 in 1000 live births and that of fetal alcohol effects 3 per 1000 live births.[10]

Although case reports of fetal alcohol syndrome from many countries of the world soon followed the original reports in the mid-1970s, case studies from Britain were notably absent. It is only in the last few years that reports of the syndrome have appeared from the United Kingdom. These studies indicate that at least in some areas of Britain the syndrome may be a significant problem. The earliest and, to date, largest study in Britain came from Beattie and co-workers in Glasgow,[11] who identified and studied forty children with the syndrome. This was soon followed by reports from Liverpool[12] (five cases) and Belfast[13] (ten cases of the syndrome, ten cases of effects). Cases of fetal alcohol syndrome do occur sporadically in other parts of Britain, but these three regions appear to be the main problem areas. It can hardly be a coincidence that in these areas poor socioeconomic conditions are combined with traditionally high levels of alcohol abuse. These reports point to an overall incidence in the United Kingdom lower than 1 in 1000 live births.

Moderate Maternal Drinking and its Effect on the Fetus

There has been growing concern that moderate or even social levels of drinking during pregnancy might be detrimental to the embryo and fetus. It becomes extremely important as well as difficult, however, to separate the effects of alcohol from other factors such as smoking, socioeconomic status, parity, and ethnic background, since all these may have a bearing on the outcome of pregnancy.

At present, there is no conclusive evidence that alcohol ingestion at moderate levels, that is less than 10 units per week (80 g), at the time of conception or during pregnancy results in an adverse fetal outcome. Moira Plant's careful analysis of over 1000 women followed prospectively during pregnancy showed quite clearly that alcohol consumption of less than 10 units in a maximum drinking week was not a cause of fetal harm, but that tobacco smoking and illegal drugs were its main predictors.[14] There may be a small effect on birthweight not only of maternal[15] but also of paternal[16] drinking. Further studies are in progress both in the USA and in Europe in an attempt to define more clearly the potential effects of such drinking. Until this information is available, it is probably sensible for women planning a pregnancy or currently pregnant, to abstain from alcohol, or at least to restrict their consumption to an occasional drink, especially in the early stages of pregnancy.

Alcohol in Breast Milk

The alcohol content of breast milk closely parallels its concentration in the mother's blood. But even if the breast milk drunk by a baby carries as much as 120 mg alcohol per 100 ml, the baby's blood concentration would still be less than 10 mg per 100 ml. An occasional drink by the mother before breast feeding will not harm the baby.[17]

The Infant and School Child

Acute Intoxication

Most paediatric departments admit a number of children each year suffering from acute alcohol intoxication.[18] Such cases fall within two relatively clear-cut age groups: toddlers who poison themselves and schoolchildren experimenting with alcohol.

Young children drink alcohol in the same way that they ingest other available medicinal or non-medicinal substances. Such incidents usually result from parental underestimation of the physical capacity of determined, inquisitive young children to explore their environment and to sample any substance they encounter. While most parents are aware that they should keep medicinal products well out of harm's way, alcoholic drinks are often left easily available to children, perhaps because parents perceive them as relatively innocuous. In addition, young children tend to copy their parents' activities. The classic scenario resulting in a drunken pre-school child is the 'Sunday morning syndrome'.[19] Parents drinking late on a Saturday night go to bed leaving bottles easily accessible. The following morning, while the parents sleep off the previous evening's excesses, their toddler finds the bottles and drinks the contents.

Older children who get drunk form a significant proportion of hospital admissions of children under fifteen years with alcohol intoxication. Most incidents are the result of experimentation or bravado in boys who underestimate the effects of what they drink. Unlike the pre-school child, many episodes occur away from the parental home and hypothermia and accidents in relation to the subsequent drunkenness may occur. In addition, the drunkenness may be part of a generalized behaviour disorder.

The Effects of Alcohol on the Child

The younger the child the higher the blood level of alcohol from a given amount of alcohol ingested. In addition, children may drink surprisingly large amounts of alcohol over very short periods of time, though their capacity to metabolize alcohol may be relatively limited due to the low level of hepatic alcohol dehydrogenase activity.[20]

Hypothermia is common in severely intoxicated children, probably arising from disordered thermoregulation induced by alcohol and aggravated by the relatively high surface area:weight ratio of the child.

Respiratory depression may occur in severely intoxicated children. They should therefore be managed in units with sufficient staff to allow close observation and with facilities for skilled intubation and respiratory support, should this prove necessary.

Hypoglycaemia is a serious complication of the 'Sunday morning syndrome'.[19] It is caused by inhibition of hepatic glucose production and is particularly liable to occur in toddlers whose liver glycogen stores are easily depleted by overnight fasting.[21]

The Effects on Children of Heavy Drinking by Parents

The scientific literature on the effects of parental alcohol abuse on the development of their children is still relatively sparse. The available evidence suggests, not surprisingly, that alcohol abuse in parents is detrimental to their children. The majority of studies have concentrated on the influence of the father's rather than the mother's drinking. Maternal drinking might seem a more serious detrimental influence on the child, but there is no available evidence to support this view. In addition, many women who drink are married to men who also have drinking problems,[27] while the converse is not always the case. Children of such families are also likely to be exposed to the marital disharmony which often accompanies (and in some cases pre-dates) heavy drinking by the parents. Inconsistent behaviour on the part of the drinking parent, perhaps with periods of over-attentiveness alternating with periods of rejection, the stress of the domestic situation, and the fear of potential or actual parental separation, must all disrupt the emotional and social development of such children. In addition, they may have to fend for themselves during periods of parental drinking, older children assuming responsibility for younger siblings. Despite these pressures, the child may help to maintain the outward facade of family 'normality' and may be loath to confide in acquaintances or school teachers. Such children often have difficulty in making and maintaining friendships, although older children may find the emotional support they lack in the family in strong peer group ties, even if this means indulging in delinquent behaviour. However, some children appear unaffected by these disturbances. Not surprisingly, the coping ability of the non-drinking parent may be crucial in modifying the effects on the child.[28]

Development and Behaviour of Children of Heavily Drinking Parents

The physical and psychological characteristics of 229 children (113 boys, 116 girls) aged 4–12 years from 141 families in which the fathers were alcohol abusers were described by Nylander in 1960;[33] 29 per cent of the children demonstrated emotional disturbances compared with only 5 per cent of matched controls. Twenty years later, Rydelius[34] assessed the social adjustment and health status of these same children. Sons of heavily drinking fathers were more likely to have non-specific medical complaints, psychiatric illness (especially alcohol and drug abuse), and social maladjustment than the controls.

Hyperactive children

Morrison and Stewart[35] found that 20 per cent of the fathers and 5 per cent of the mothers of 59 hyperactive children were alcohol abusers, compared with 10 per cent of the fathers and none of the mothers of 41 control children. Twelve parents of hyperactive children had been hyperactive themselves and half were excessive drinkers in later life. The association between hyperactivity and fetal exposure to alcohol has already been described (p. 93).

Juvenile delinquency

Juvenile delinquency seems to be more common in children, especially boys, of parents who abuse alcohol. It may be related to significant alcohol abuse in these young people themselves. Drinking patterns of 500 male delinquents aged 7–20 years in Massachusetts,[36] showed that 13 per cent were 'heavy drinkers' while 10 per cent were 'addictive drinkers'. Such young people have often lost one or both parents in early life, have spent part of their youth in institutional care and begin drinking at an early age. Psychiatric and emotional problems also appear to be increased in children and adolescents of such parents, and both drug addiction and anorexia nervosa are reported to be associated with heavy parental drinking.

Child Abuse

Alcoholism has been associated with an increased level of child abuse.[29,30] However, in a recent survey by the National Society for the Prevention of Cruelty to Children of trends in child abuse in the United Kingdom, persistent misuse of alcohol does not feature as a significant provoking factor.[31] Alcohol intoxication rather than alcoholism may be the relevant factor.[32]

Adolescents

Most children are likely to come into contact with alcohol, directly or indirectly, at a young age. Their early understanding of its effects and their concept of its use initially reflect parental attitudes and drinking habits. Later, peer influence and that of society at large become increasingly important as young people progress through late childhood and adolescence. Surprisingly, British teenagers have a much higher level of alcohol experience than their contemporaries in the USA.[21-23]

However, while problems of chronic ingestion of alcohol may begin in adolescence, the short-term physical effect of alcohol on the health of schoolchildren appears at present to be slight. Over the age of fifteen years, alcohol use appears less and less an experimental event and regular drinkers become increasingly at risk of injury or death from alcohol-related accidents or violence. The frequency of alcohol abuse quickly rises during the mid and late teens. Although predominantly involving males, it is seen increasingly among young women in recent years.[24] This is worrying, for while most problem drinking in young men seems to be resolved to some extent with time, problem drinking among young women may well become a permanent pattern.[25] It is reflected in an increase in recent years in drunkenness and 'drinking and driving' convictions in young women.[26]

References

1. Lilly, L.J. (1975) Investigations, *In Vitro* and *In Vivo*, of the Effects of Disulfiram (Antabuse) on Human Lymphocyte Chromosomes. *Toxicology* 4: 331–40.
2. Kaufman, M.H. (1983) Ethanol-Induced Chromosomal Abnormalities at Conception. *Nature* 302: 258–60.
3. Sokol, R.J., Miller, S.I., and Reed, G. (1980) Alcohol Abuse During Pregnancy: an Epidemiological Study. *Alcoholism: Clinical and Experimental Research* (New York) 4: 135–45.
4. Clarren, S.K. and Smith, D.W. (1978) The Fetal Alcohol Syndrome. *New England Journal of Medicine* 298: 1063–067.
5. Rosett, H.L. (1980) A Clinical Perspective on the Fetal Alcohol Syndrome. *Alcoholism: Clinical and Experimental Research* (New York) 4: 119–22.
6. Beattie, J.O., Day, R.E., Cockburn, F., and Garg, R.A. (1983) Alcohol and the Fetus in the West of Scotland. *British Medical Journal* 287: 17–20.
7. Streissguth, A.P., Herman, C.S., and Smith, D. (1978) Intelligence, Behavior and Dysmorphogenesis in the Fetal Alcohol Syndrome: a Report on 20 Clinical Cases. *Journal of Pediatrics* 92: 363–67.
8. Clarren, S.K., Alvord, E.C., Sumi, S.M., and Streissguth, A.P. (1978) Brain Malformations Related to Prenatal Exposure to Ethanol. *Journal of Pediatrics* 92: 64–7.
9. Spiegel, P.G., Pekman, W.M., Rich, H.B., Versteeg, C.N., Nelson, V., and Dudnikov, M. (1979) The Orthopaedic Aspects of the Fetal

Alcohol Syndrome. *Clinical Orthopaedics and Related Research* 139: 58–63.

10. Abel, E.L. (1984) *Fetal Alcohol Syndrome and Fetal Alcohol Effects.* New York: Plenum Press, pp. 73–82.

11. Beattie, J.O., Day, R.E., and Cockburn, F. (1981) Fetal Alcohol Syndrome: 40 Cases from the West of Scotland. Abstract. Exeter: Paediatric Research Society.

12. Poskitt, E.M.E., Hensey, O.J., and Smith, C.S. (1982) Alcohol, Other Drugs and the Fetus. *Developmental Medicine and Child Neurology* 24: 596–602.

13. Halliday, H.L., Reid, M.McC., and McLure, G. (1982) Results of Heavy Drinking in Pregnancy. *British Journal of Obstetrics and Gynaecology* 89: 892–95.

14. Plant, M. (1985) *Women, Drinking, and Pregnancy.* London: Tavistock Publications.

15. Mills, J.L., Graubard, B.I., Harley, E.E., Rhoads, G.G., and Berends, H.W. (1984) Maternal Alcohol Consumption and Birthweight. *Journal of the American Medical Association* 252: 1875–879.

16. Little, R.E. and Sing, C.F. (1986) Association of Father's Drinking and Infant's Birthweight. *New England Journal of Medicine* 314: 1644.

17. Laurton, M.E. (1985) Alcohol in Breast Milk. *Australia and New Zealand Journal of Obstetrics and Gynaecology* 25: 71–3.

18. Beattie, J.O., Hull, D., and Cockburn, F. (1985) Children Acutely Intoxicated with Alcohol in Glasgow and Nottingham 1973–1985. Abstract. St Andrews: Paediatric Research Society.

19. Bradford, D.E. (1979) Alcohol Related Hypoglycaemia in Children Again – a Sunday Morning Hazard? *British Journal of Alcohol and Alcoholism* 14: 84–5.

20. Pikkarainen, P.H. and Raiha, N.C.R. (1969) Development of Alcohol Dehydrogenase Activity in the Human Liver. *Nature* 222: 563–64.

21. Gillam, D.M. and Harper, J.R. (1973) Hypoglycaemia After Alcohol Ingestion. *Lancet* 1: 829–30.

22. Hawker, A. (1978) *Adolescents and Alcohol.* London: Edsell.

23. Plant, M.A., Peck, D.F., and Stuart, R. (1982) Self-Reported Drinking Habits and Alcohol-Related Consequences Amongst a Cohort of Scottish Teenagers. *British Journal of Addiction* 77: 75–90.

24. Shaw, S. (1980) The Causes of Increasing Drink Problems Amongst Women. In *Women and Alcohol.* London: Tavistock Publications, pp. 1–40.

25. Smart, R.G., Gray, G., and Bennett, C. (1978) Predictors of Drinking and Signs of Heavy Drinking Among High School Students. *International Journal of Addiction* 13: 1079–094.

26. McNeill, A. (1983) Alcohol Problems: Trends and Prospects. Paper presented at a symposium on Alcohol and Child Development. London: Institute of Alcohol Studies.

27. Jacob, T., Favorini, A., Meisel, S.S., and Anderson, C.M. (1978) The Alcoholic's Spouse, Children and Family Interaction. *Journal of the Study of Alcohol* 39: 1231–251.

28. Wilson, C. and Orford, J. (1978) Children of Alcoholics. *Journal of the Study of Alcohol* 39: 121–42.
29. Mayer, J. and Black, R. (1977) The Relationship Between Alcoholism and Child Abuse and Neglect. In F. A. Seixas (ed.) *Currents in Alcoholism, Vol. 2. Psychiatric, Social and Epidemiological Studies.* New York: Grune and Stratton.
30. Smith, S.M., Hanson, R., and Noble, S. (1974) Social Aspects of the Battered Baby Syndrome. *British Journal of Psychiatry* 125: 568–82.
31. Creighton, S.J. (1984) *Trends in Child Abuse, 1977–1982.* London: National Society for the Prevention of Cruelty to Children (NSPCC).
32. Gil, D.G. (1968) California Pilot Study. In R. C. Helfer and C. H. Kempe (eds) *The Battered Child.* Chicago: University of Chicago Press, pp. 215–25.
33. Nylander, I. (1960) Children of Alcoholic Fathers. *Acta Paediatrica Scandinavica* 49: 1–134.
34. Rydelius, P.A. (1981) Children of Alcoholic Fathers. Their Social Adjustment and Their Health Status over 20 Years. *Acta Paediatrica Scandinavica* Suppl. 286: 1–89.
35. Morrison, J.R. and Stewart, M.A. (1971) A Family Study of the Hyperactive Child Syndrome. *Biological Psychiatry* 3: 189–95.
36. MacKay, J.R. (1961) Clinical Observations on Adolescent Problem Drinkers. *Quarterly Journal of Studies on Alcohol* 22: 124–34.

14

MEDICAL RESPONSIBILITIES

Summary

Physicians have an important part to play in reducing the harm done by alcohol. In their daily work they must become better able to detect alcohol-related problems, and to detect them at an earlier stage. At the moment their role is too often concerned with managing serious physical damage. Earlier detection should lead to more preventive work and more effective treatment. The second task for physicians is to take a lead in informing other doctors and professionals and the public about alcohol-related problems. Third, physicians must impress on government that political measures may be necessary to reduce the extensive damage caused in our society by alcohol.

The Physician's Role in Combating Alcohol-Associated Damage

This report has detailed the harm that alcohol can do to physical health and has shown that most systems of the body can be damaged. The psychological, family, social, and economic problems associated with alcohol have also been mentioned and are in many ways more important than the physical health problems. No previous report from Britain has looked so comprehensively at the harm done to physical health, but many other reports (see p. 2) – most recently the second one from the Royal College of Psychiatrists[1] – have considered other aspects.[2,3,4] Most have made recommendations on how the damage may be reduced, and the most comprehensive strategy was produced by the Scottish Health Education Coordinating Committee.[2] Recognizing the wide range of problems associated with alcohol, it directed detailed recommendations to most sections of Scottish society, including all types of doctors. Most of the recommendations could apply equally well to England and Northern

Ireland and a similar strategy has already been suggested for Wales.[3] We are impressed by both the Scottish and the Welsh reports and support their recommendations. A practical guide for action for use by lay or professional people to prevent alcohol problems has been published recently by Tether and Robinson.[4]

Our recommendations are directed primarily towards physicians, who have a responsibility beyond that to their individual patients. Physicians also have a role to play in educating other professionals and the public on alcohol problems and in impressing on government the need for political action to reduce alcohol-associated harm.

The Physician's Role with Patients

Detection

By the time medical advice is sought about alcohol abuse, it is often too late to reverse the damage or break the dependence, although progressive deterioration may be halted if the patient can be persuaded to stop drinking. Present methods of treatment at this stage are seldom successful in more than a quarter of patients[5] and greater emphasis needs to be placed on prevention. At present, no more than one in ten drinkers is identified by most surveillance programmes and the difficulties of early detection should not be underestimated.[6] Heavy drinkers are not likely to consult health care workers; there is no consensus as to what constitutes safe drinking;[7] and there is a general lack of awareness (together with denial) among many lay people and health professionals as to what are the danger signals. Even when the doctor is involved, he or she may not appreciate the significance of the symptoms because they mimic many common diseases; sometimes it is members of the family rather than the heavy drinker who come for treatment.

It is often difficult to obtain a proper drinking history; people seem unwilling to answer questions about alcohol in the way they will about cigarette smoking or drugs. We recommend that:

- **Every person seen in general practice or in hospital should be asked about his or her alcohol intake as a matter of routine, along with questions about smoking and medication, and the answers recorded.**

Information regarding quantity and frequency of drinking are the minimum requirements; the answers may be only approximate, but an idea of the importance of drinking to the individual can be obtained with experience.

People who say they do not drink at all may be teetotal or reformed drinkers. The individual who states he only has 'a few' may be concealing a heavy intake, and those who admit they used to drink heavily but do not drink much now may still be suffering from the effects of excessive drinking.

Certain presentations should always raise suspicion of alcohol abuse: chest pain in young to middle-aged men, often accompanied by palpitations, shortness of breath and anxiety, with a normal electrocardiograph; abdominal pain mimicking peptic ulcer; and psychoneurotic symptoms. Problem drinkers are often admitted to hospital with chest pain, rib fractures, abdominal pain, fits, 'concussion', and trauma, without the underlying alcohol problem being recognized. The elderly is a group in which alcohol abuse is underestimated because covert, excessive drinking may be a response to loneliness, depression, and loss of mental faculties, which may in turn lead to malnutrition and social difficulties. Increased sensitivity to relatively small amounts of alcohol may contribute to confusion, falls, injuries, and heart failure.

Physicians should recognize the plethoric, moon-shaped face of the chronic drinker, and should consider alcohol excess when they first see a patient with raised blood pressure, glycosuria, or gout. They, and especially general practitioners, should take more notice of the social concomitants of heavy drinking; problems with marriage, work, and the law may be confided to the doctor by parties other than the heavy drinker. The present reluctance of doctors to become involved helps neither patient nor profession.

Information about the pattern of drinking in different populations, for example rural versus inner city, is scanty. Instead of responding solely to patients' needs, we recommend that:

● **Doctors should take the lead in defining drinking habits in their practice by means of questionnaires, breath alcohol measurements and blood tests.**[8]

For example, simple questionnaires about alcohol incorporated in general health histories about eating, smoking, and taking exercise could be given to a sample of patients in a practice. Special questionnaires designed to detect problem drinkers like CAGE and brief MAST could then be used for case finding.

The use of an alcolmeter to test for breath alcohol (100 mg/100 ml at any time indicates heavy drinking) has been described in general practice;[9] its use could well be extended to hospitals. Biochemical (gamma-glutamyl transferase (GGT), fasting triglycerides, and urates) and haematological (mean corpuscular volume, MCV) tests have been widely used in detecting heavy drinkers, but their value has been questioned;[6,10] like all investigations, they should be used to support other evidence rather than in isolation. Moreover, figures for heavy drinkers may be within the normal range, but the spread tends to be skewed towards the upper end for MCV, GGT, triglycerides, and urates and towards the lower end in the case of blood urea. It is likely that the use of a number of tests could produce an index of suspicion of heavy drinking: a combination of questionnaire and blood tests, for example, improves the accuracy of detection.[11] Individuals at risk should be encouraged to use a drinking diary[12] which may alert them to dangerous levels of drinking.

Management

At present, a disproportionate amount of time and money is devoted to the medical treatment of a small proportion of individuals with severe alcohol-related problems, and the generally poor results have led people to question the value of medical treatment. Most alcohol-associated problems arise in the community and are increasingly dealt with by alliances of health professionals other than doctors, and by voluntary workers. Doctors need to develop greater awareness of how commonly alcohol underlies the problems for which their patients consult them, in hospital as well as in general practice. If they treat only the presenting problem they lose a valuable opportunity not only to protect the individual from further harm but also to educate people about alcohol.

Advice is most likely to be effective if it is given to heavy drinkers before they have developed problems or become dependent.[13,14] Evidence is accumulating that simple advice about cutting down drinking given by a doctor or other health worker is effective in as many as two-thirds of heavy drinkers. If necessary, continued support can be provided by counselling, the use of a diary card,[12] and joining a group such as Drinkwatchers.

Problem and dependent drinkers need to abstain completely and alcohol (and sometimes drugs) must be replaced by long-term support and counselling. The outlook is improved if help is available from family and employer. A short period of hospitalization may be required during which decisions can be taken about referral to other specialists, long-term residential care, attendance at meetings of Alcoholics Anonymous (AA), and the support needed on return to the community.

Most alcohol problems can be managed by a community alcohol team. We strongly support:

- **The setting up of community alcohol teams.**

They have the advantage of providing a variety of services which can be tailored to the needs of individual clients. They are able to respond to local crises, keep in touch with the client, and act as a focus of awareness about alcohol in the locality. To be effective they need a considerable range of health workers, including social workers, community psychiatric nurses, counsellors, district nurses, and health visitors, as well as volunteers such as reformed alcoholics. They must have close contacts with occupational health nurses, the probation service, welfare organizations, the church, and local schools. Medical representation should include interested general practitioners and hospital physicians or psychiatrists. A health district with a population of 2–300,000 would have a potential clientele of 10–15,000 individuals. Medical expertise should be provided by a physician or psychiatrist with an interest in alcohol problems. We suggest that:

- **Not more than four to six hospital beds would be required for short stay, emergency treatment and they should be immediately available (other demands being equal) for admission of alcohol abusers.**

It is important to emphasize that these beds are not just for drying out but so that individuals can be removed temporarily and rapidly from their environment at times of stress. Hospital staff should be able to respond not only to requests from general practitioners but from members of the community alcohol team, voluntary bodies like the alcoholism councils, AA and ACCEPT, and from drinkers themselves and their relatives and friends.

The successful functioning of the hospital unit depends on rapid assessment (and hence turnover), early and clear decisions on management of patients, and close liaison with members of the community alcohol team. It should also act as a source of information and advice, as well as training health workers about alcohol and its problems. It should be able to carry out research and also particularly evaluation of its own treatment programme.

The Physician's Role in Education

The first group who need education on alcohol problems are medical students and young doctors. The performance of young doctors in obtaining an alcohol history is poor.[15] During undergraduate training emphasis should be placed on all the problems arising from excessive alcohol drinking rather than just its physical effects. We recommend that:

- **Integrated modules involving experts from disciplines other than medicine could be taught in both the pre-clinical and clinical courses.**[16,17]

New initiatives are needed to educate established doctors in detection and prevention of alcohol problems and in counselling. Local medical expertise will be required in developing community alcohol teams; in addition to psychiatrists, interested general practitioners, community physicians, and general physicians should be trained in alcohol problems. Physicians could be recruited from gastroenterologists, clinical pharmacologists, and clinical epidemiologists, and from junior staff engaged in liaison work or research in alcohol and addiction problems. Doctors must recognize too that their own profession is particularly at risk from alcohol abuse. Individual doctors should examine their own drinking, and the whole profession should consider trying to reduce its alcohol consumption. This should lead to an unequivocal reduction in cirrhosis and other measures of alcohol damage among doctors, which might impress on the public its own need to reduce alcohol consumption. The model here is the way that doctors reduced their smoking and so their lung cancer death rates.

Education by example is one way in which doctors can convey to the public the risks of alcohol. In addition, they should help in promoting drinking in moderation as part of a programme that includes advice about diet, drugs, smoking, and exercise. They should make sure that information about alcohol is available in clinics and surgeries.

On a broader canvas, doctors should encourage a shift in public attitudes from the view that drunkenness is something to be treated as a joke, and that those who do not drink or only drink moderately are somehow abnormal. People frequently remark that it is almost impossible to say no when offered an alcoholic drink in a situation where alcohol is usually drunk, for example, at parties, lunches, or in pubs. Pressures are such (ridicule, imitation, bravado, conformity) that if society does not make it easier to refuse, the toll in alcohol problems will continue. It is encouraging to note the increasing availability and acceptability of non-alcoholic drinks (a trend particularly apparent in the USA) as alternatives to alcohol.

All levels of society need to develop a better understanding of the dangers of alcohol. This will require improved school education and instruction of the young by parental example. Rather than doctors and other educators simply spelling out the potential dangers of alcohol, more emphasis needs to be placed on teaching general life skills such as assertiveness and resisting peer pressure, and on developing self-esteem. This can be complemented later by instruction in 'safe' drinking.

One group of doctors who may have particular opportunities to influence education on alcohol are occupational physicians. Many of the larger corporations, like the Post Office, already have alcohol policies which cover the use of alcohol at work, education on alcohol issues, and markers (like diminished work performance) which may be used to assist in the early identification of drink problems. We recommend that:

- **Occupational physicians should encourage the corporations with which they are associated to adopt comprehensive alcohol policies.**

Advice on 'Safe' Limits

One part of public education for which doctors should be particularly responsible is in advising on the 'safe' limits of alcohol consumption. Unfortunately there is insufficient scientific evidence to make completely confident statements on how much alcohol is 'safe'. Safety is a compound of individual vulnerability and the circumstances in which drinking takes place. It is essential, however, that this is not used as an excuse for inaction, since doctors and patients need guidance which is easily understood and reasonable. While recognizing that more research is needed to define 'safe' drinking, we put forward the following recommendations:

- **Individuals who drink alcohol regularly should attempt to keep their intake within 'safe limits'.**

- **We define *safe* levels as up to 21 units a week for men and up to 14 units a week for women. At such levels most individuals are unlikely to come to any harm, provided the total amount** is not drunk in one or two bouts and that there are occasional drink-free days.

- Drinking becomes *hazardous* between 21–49 units a week for men and 14–35 units for women. Individuals in this category should be able to reduce their intake to safe levels when the dangers are pointed out. They can be encouraged to keep drinking diaries and to attend groups like Drinkwatchers; they should be able to call on support from doctors and other health workers.

- Levels above 49 units a week for men and 35 units for women are *dangerous*. Individuals who persistently exceed them require help from health care workers, voluntary bodies like Alcoholics Anonymous, or specialist alcohol agencies. They should on no account be encouraged to continue by collusion or covering up by family, friends, or colleagues, otherwise it may be too late to help.

Physicians, Government, and Alcohol Problems

Health and education professionals cannot reduce alcohol damage dramatically themselves. Evidence reviewed earlier (Chapter 2, p. 23) suggests that while alcohol consumption remains high in Britain damage will also remain high. All of the previous reports on alcohol that we have mentioned[1,2,3,4] have taken the view that at the very least the government should try to prevent alcohol consumption rising any further. We take this view as well. Indeed, we are convinced that a reduction would be good for the health of Britain. We recommend that:

- The annual consumption of alcohol should not be allowed to rise above the present level of 8 litres per head (equivalent to 3 units a day) and that steps should be taken by both public and government to reduce annual consumption to about 5 litres (or 2 units a day) per head over the next ten years.

The most effective way in which government can change consumption is by manipulating the price of alcohol. The price has for a long time been unrealistically low, and the failure to increase taxes in the 1986 budget was a particular blow to those of us who daily confront the results of Britain's high alcohol consumption. The government should look carefully at the extensive evidence that suggests that steady increases in the real price of alcohol will lead to a drop in consumption, which in its turn will lead to a fall in alcohol associated harm of all types. We recommend that:

- **The real price of alcohol be increased over the next five to ten years.**

The importance of advertising in influencing alcohol consumption is less clear. While further research on the relation between advertising and consumption is likely to prove inconclusive, we recommend that:

- **More stringent rules for alcohol advertising should be formulated to protect the young who are particularly vulnerable.**

We also recommend that:

- **Sponsorship of sport and the arts by the liquor industry should be restricted.**

The linking of alcohol advertisements with sporting events seems particularly wrong. We recommend that:

- **The government consider carefully the case for requiring all alcoholic drinks to show the quantity of alcohol on the container in simple measures that the average individual can understand.**

Units or grams of alcohol are preferable to the present weight per volume or proof measure. This is particularly important for beer, which comes in a variety of strengths. We recommend that:

- **A much tougher stance should be adopted on 'drinking and driving' which is responsible for an unacceptably high number of injuries and deaths (see Chapter 12).**

We would particularly urge the government to look at practices in Scandinavian countries where it is now accepted that people do not drive if they are expecting to drink. We unreservedly deplore the granting of licenses to garages to sell alcohol. We hope the government will back the production of an alcohol sensor which will make it impossible to start a car if the breath alcohol is above a pre-set level.

Drinking at sporting events such as football, and under-age drinking, especially in public houses, should be discouraged. Police and probation services need to be encouraged to refer drinking offenders for treatment and rehabilitation.

The debate on liberalizing licensing hours has not yet reached a firm conclusion but the increase in the number of outlets, such as supermarkets and off-licences, as well as the availability of home-brew kits, has contributed to the rising consumption especially in the home. The ability to buy alcohol at any time on trains, aeroplanes, and ferries not only encourages consumption but contributes to inappropriate drinking in public. Prohibition of drinking in public places and on public transport such as buses and tubes, might well be acceptable to the public. We recommend that:

- **The government should not yet take steps that would liberalize the licensing laws and make alcohol more readily available.**

The government, we recommend:

- **Should provide more money from the tax on alcoholic drinks for education and research on alcohol problems, and operational research especially devoted to detection and prevention should be encouraged.**

The government should support Action on Alcohol Abuse (Triple A) to stimulate a continuing debate on the control of alcohol abuse in the same way that it does Action on Smoking and Health (ASH).

It was suggested by the government's own Central Policy Review Staff in 1979 that a single policy body was needed to coordinate the work of the sixteen government departments currently concerned with alcohol.

An inter-departmental committee on drug abuse has recently been set up but, although alcohol abuse is considerably more serious in terms of the number of people affected, no comparable body exists to deal with this important problem. We recommend that:

- **A single government body be formed to coordinate all aspects of alcohol use and abuse.**

The alarming rise in alcohol consumption throughout the world, and particularly in Third World countries, is of concern to us as physicians. Brewing companies see these Third World countries in terms of export markets to be exploited; we would ask that the wider public health issues and moral arguments be taken into account.

References

1. Royal College of Psychiatrists (1986) *Alcohol: Our Favourite Drug.* London: Tavistock Publications.

2. Scottish Health Education Coordinating Committee (1985) *Health Education in the Prevention of Alcohol Related Problems*. Edinburgh: SHECC.
3. Health Education Advisory Committee for Wales (1986) *Dealing with Alcohol Problems in Wales*. Cardiff: HEAC.
4. Tether, P. and Robinson, D. (1986) *Preventing Alcohol Problems: A Guide to Local Action*. London: Tavistock Publications.
5. Valliant, G.E., Clark, W., Cyprus, C., Milofsky, E.S., Kopp, J., Wulsin, V.N., and Mogielnicki, N.P. (1983) Prospective Study of Alcoholism Treatment. Eight-Year Follow-Up. *American Journal of Medicine* 75: 455–63.
6. Leading article (1980) Screening Tests for Alcoholism? *Lancet* ii: 117–18.
7. Anderson, P., Cremona, A., and Wallace, P. (1984) What Are Safe Levels of Alcohol Consumption? *British Medical Journal* 289: 165–68.
8. Various authors (1982) Alcohol Problems. London: British Medical Journal.
9. Wiseman, S.M., Tomson, P.V., Barnett, J.M., Jenns, M., and Wilton, J. (1982) Use of an Alcolmeter to Detect Problem Drinkers. *British Medical Journal* 285: 1089–090.
10. Chick, J., Kreitman, N., and Plant, M. (1981) Mean Cell Volume and Gamma-Glutamyl Transpeptidase as Markers of Drinking in Working Men. *Lancet* i: 1249–251.
11. Bernadt, M.W., Mumford, J., Taylor, C., Smith, B., and Murray, R.M. (1982) Comparison of Questionnaire and Laboratory Tests in the Detection of Excessive Drinking and Alcoholism. *Lancet* i: 325–28.
12. Grant, M. (1984) *Same Again. A Guide to Safer Drinking*. Harmondsworth: Penguin.
13. Chick, J. (1982) Do Alcoholics Recover? *British Medical Journal* 285: 3–4.
14. Skinner, H.A. and Holt, S. (1983) Early Intervention for Alcohol Problems. *Journal of the Royal College of General Practitioners* 33: 78–91.
15. Barrison, I.G., Viola, L., and Murray-Lyon, I.M. (1980) Do Housemen Take an Adequate History? *British Medical Journal* 281: 1040.
16. Skinner, H.A., Holt, S., and Israel, Y. (1981) Early Identification of Alcohol Abuse. 1. Critical Issues and Psychosocial Indications for a Composite Index. *Canadian Medical Association Journal* 124: 1141–152.
17. Holt, S., Skinner, H.A., and Israel, Y. (1981) Early Identification of Alcohol Abuse. 2. Clinical and Laboratory Indications. *Canadian Medical Association Journal* 124: 1279–299.

APPENDIX 1

Alcohol Metabolism

Blood levels

Drinking a unit of alcohol (half a pint of beer, a glass of wine, or a single pub measure of spirits) increases the blood alcohol level within the first hour by about 15 mg/100 ml in a man and by nearly 20 mg/100 ml in a woman because of her smaller body size and relatively smaller body water content.

In a healthy person alcohol is cleared from the blood by the liver at a rate of about 15 mg/100 ml an hour. Thus, if somebody's blood alcohol level is 100 mg/100 ml, it will still be above the legal limit for driving (80 mg/100 ml) more than an hour later and for 3–4 hours will remain at levels which expose the individual to significant risk of having an accident (*Figure 9*). It will be six hours before the blood is once again completely free of alcohol and may take even longer in someone whose liver is damaged or who is taking medicinal or other drugs which interfere with the metabolism of alcohol.

Metabolism of ethanol

This section is concerned with the metabolism of ethanol[1,2] as this is the alcohol present in alcoholic beverages.

Oxidation

The liver is the principal site of ethanol metabolism. The first step is oxidation to acetaldehyde and hydrogen by three separate oxidizing systems (*Figure 9*). Alcohol dehydrogenase (ADH) accounts for the majority of ethanol oxidation; the remainder is oxidized by the microsomal enzyme oxidizing system (MEOS). The activity of

MEOS may be increased by several drugs and by chronic alcohol abuse and this may be the reason for the increased drug and ethanol tolerance in heavy drinkers. A third, and in normal circumstances qualitatively unimportant oxidative pathway, is mediated by the enzyme catalase.

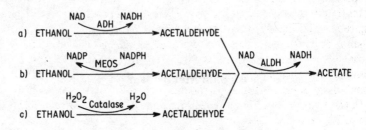

Figure 9 The metabolism of ethanol.

Abbreviations: ADH: Alcohol dehydrogenase
                  ALDH: Aldehyde dehydrogenase
                  MEOS: Microsomal enzyme-oxidizing system
                  NAD: Coenzyme I
                  NADP: Coenzyme II
                  H_2O_2: Hydrogen peroxide

Acetaldehyde, one of the products of ethanol oxidation, is a highly toxic substance and is itself removed by oxidation via the enzyme aldehyde dehydrogenase (ALDH) which is widely distributed in many body tissues. The activity of this enzyme plays an important role in determining the concentration of this toxic compound and so the degree and site of cell damage. ALDH exists in several isoenzyme forms whose activity and distribution are under genetic control and this probably plays an important part in determining the susceptibility of individuals to acetaldehyde-related tissue damage and perhaps also to alcohol addiction.

The products of acetaldehyde oxidation are acetate, which is rapidly and safely metabolized further to acetate, and yet more hydrogen ions. The production of hydrogen ions in these oxidizing reactions profoundly affects many of the cell's metabolic activities. They react with the co-enzymes NAD and NADP and so shift the oxidization-reduction potential of the cell. This results, among other changes, in alterations of steroid metabolism and in a decrease of glucose synthesis in the liver.

Cell damage

Ethanol can injure all tissues and systems of the body. It does this both directly and through its metabolic products; in addition, secondary damage may arise because of an immunological reaction to ethanol-damaged cell membranes. The toxicity of ethanol is potentiated by malnutrition, vitamin deficiency, drug abuse, and cigarette smoking, frequent findings in heavy drinkers. Conversely, ethanol enhances the action of cancer-promoting agents, including those of cigarette smoke. It also changes the metabolism of many drugs and medicines while they themselves may affect the metabolism of ethanol and enhance its damaging effect.

In the liver, acetaldehyde interferes with cell respiration, damages the cell's internal transport systems for calcium and proteins, changes the activity of membrane-bound enzymes, and increases cell permeability with the loss of important internal constituents.

In the nervous system and brain, the acute toxic effects of ethanol metabolism are probably related to its incorporation into cell membranes. This increases their fluidity with a consequent disordering effect on the function of important proteins associated with cell membranes such as those involved in the recognition and transmission of nerve messages, and in the activity of several regulatory enzymes. Tolerance to ethanol, on the other hand, is associated with increasing rigidity of cell membranes brought about by an increase in their cholesterol and saturated fatty acid content.

In the brain, as in the heart and the pancreas, which are also prone to ethanol-induced tissue damage, little or no acetaldehyde is produced. Cell damage in these tissues may be due partly to the direct effect of ethanol and partly to non-oxidative esterification of fatty acids with ethanol. The presence of such fatty acid ethyl esters and their further metabolism, including fatty acid peroxidation with production of abnormal free-radical activity, probably plays an important role in causing selective organ damage.

Identifying the Alcohol Abuser

Laboratory tests

Many attempts have been made to devise practicable laboratory tests for the identification of individuals who drink excessively. A combination of the following tests appears to be the most useful and will identify about 70 per cent of such individuals:

1. gamma glutamyl transferase (GGT);
2. aspartate transaminase (AST);
3. uric acid;
4. triglyceride;
5. mean corpuscle volume (MCV).

However, recent studies[3,4] have shown that the most reliable indicators of alcohol abuse remain a high index of suspicion, an accurate history of drinking, and the application of a brief questionnaire on alcohol problems such as the Michigan alcoholism screening test (MAST). When these clinical investigations are backed up by laboratory tests, more than 90 per cent of individuals with alcohol problems can be identified.

References

1. Peters, T.J. (1982) Ethanol Metabolism. *British Medical Bulletin* 38: 17–20.
2. Laposata, E.A. and Lange, L.G. (1986) Presence of Monoxidative Ethanol Metabolism in Human Organs Commonly Damaged by Ethanol Abuse. *Science* 231: 497–99.
3. Wallace, P. (1986) Looking for Patients at Risk Because of Their Drinking. *Journal of the Royal Society of Medicine* 79: 129–30.
4. Skinner, H.A., Holt, S., Shen, W.J., and Israel, Y. (1986) Clinical Versus Laboratory Detection of Alcohol Abuse: the Alcohol Clinical Index. *British Medical Journal* 292: 1703–708.

APPENDIX 2

Interaction of Alcohol with Medicines

Summary

The interaction of drugs with alcohol is complex. In general, acute ingestion of drugs and alcohol enhances the effect of both substances, but in persistent drinkers, drug activity is often diminished because alcohol induces the production of enzymes which may accelerate their breakdown. Individuals with alcoholic liver disease or malnutrition may be more sensitive to the effects of certain drugs. Some drugs interfere with the breakdown of alcohol leading to the accumulation of one of its toxic products, acetaldehyde. High concentrations of this compound in the blood produce a severe adverse reaction called the Antabuse-effect. Antabuse is a drug prescribed to curb alcohol abuse which prevents individuals drinking because of the threat of the unpleasant consequences.

When alcohol and drugs are taken together each affects the other's behaviour. Their interaction is often complex and ill-understood,[1-5] so that no single mechanism is responsible for all interactions nor is the effect of an individual drug always predictable. But in general, effects can be simply classified into three broad groups:

1. the additive action of alcohol and drugs taken acutely;
2. the diminished effect of drugs in an individual who drinks regularly; and
3. the increased sensitivity to drugs conferred by malnutrition and severe liver damage, for example cirrhosis.

Acute Ingestion of Alcohol

Alcohol in more than small amounts depresses the rate of drug metabolism, so that the action of some drugs is exaggerated (*Table 11*).

This is especially important in the case of drugs which act on the central nervous system, for example dextropropoxyphene, whose depressant effect may be fatally aggravated by alcohol. The activity of all central nervous system depressants is enhanced, psychomotor performance is impaired, and patients should be warned against drinking alcohol when taking these drugs. Short-acting benzodiazepine tranquillizers, oxazepam (Oxanid), lorazepam (Ativan), are safer than diazepam (Valium).

Table 11 *Acute ingestion of alcohol*

Decreased drug breakdown causing enhanced drug activity

benzodiazepines	monoamine oxidase inhibitors
barbiturates	oral hypoglycaemic agents
phenothiazines	phenytoin
tricyclic antidepressants	warfarin
chlormethiazole	metronidazole
dextropropoxyphene	

Drugs which have strong anticholinergic properties, for example amitriptyline (Tryptizol, Lentizol), can provoke extrapyramidal symptoms if alcohol is taken. Hypertensive crises occur if patients taking monoamine oxidase inhibitors (Marplan, Nardil) drink wines with a high tyramine content.

It is less well known that drugs acting on the central nervous system depress the rate of alcohol breakdown, so that the effect of a given amount of alcohol may be exaggerated. A further paradox is that a patient's depression may be worsened if alcohol is taken during treatment with tricyclic antidepressants (Tofranil, Prothiaden). A ban on alcohol whenever drugs acting on the central nervous system are prescribed seems the only sensible way of avoiding potentially dangerous side effects.

The action of oral hypoglycaemic agents in diabetics is increased by alcohol: the hypoglycaemic effect may not be apparent for some time after alcohol has been taken. The risk of bleeding with warfarin is well known.

Drugs may affect the metabolism of alcohol: the usual result is inhibition with accumulation of acetaldehyde, though it is difficult to know how significant these actions are in clinical practice, except in the case of disulfiram (Antabuse) and chlorpropamide. Similarly, the few substances which induce (increase) alcohol metabolism, such as phenobarbitone, clofibrate, and fructose, have mostly been tested in animals in large dosage, and have as yet no practical application in speeding up the body's disposal of alcohol.

Chronic alcohol abuse

The effect of prolonged heavy alcohol consumption (and also cigarette smoking, which is indulged in by 90 per cent of heavy drinkers, and marijuana) is to increase the activity of the enzymes responsible for drug metabolism. The rate of removal of drugs by the liver is speeded up, so that their therapeutic effect may be reduced by as much as half so that normally prescribed drug dosages may not be enough; alcohol abusers often tolerate large doses of drugs (*Table 12*). Examples of the need for increased dosages are encountered in practice when treating withdrawal symptoms with chlormethiazole and benzodiazepines and thrombotic episodes with warfarin.

Table 12 *Chronic alcoholism*

Increased drug breakdown causing diminished drug activity

barbiturates	tolbutamide
meprobamate	phenytoin
benzodiazepines	warfarin
chlormethaziole	paracetamol
anitipyrine	alkylating agents

Malnutrition in chronic alcohol abusers should be borne in mind as a possible, though uncommon, cause of increased sensitivity to drugs, since a low protein, high carbohydrate intake with deficient minerals and vitamins will depress many enzyme systems and impair drug metabolism.

People who drink to excess frequently abuse drugs, just as some drug addicts become dependent on alcohol; it is difficult to provide figures but perhaps one in ten alcohol abusers also abuse drugs. The most common combinations are with chlormethiazole, benzodiazepines, barbiturates, and dextropropoxyphene. Lethal interactions between alcohol and relatively small doses of these drugs have been recorded. Cross dependency between alcohol and benzodiazepines or chlormethiazole can sometimes arise.

Some drugs interfere with the metabolism of alcohol by competing for enzymes. This is the basis of the Antabuse reaction, used in the treatment of alcohol abuse; other drugs can cause a similar reaction

Table 13 *Antabuse reaction*

disulfiram	sulphonylureas
calcium carbimide	chloramphenicol
metronidazole	furazolidone
griseofulvin	mepacrine
procarbazine	chloral hydrate

(*Table 13*). Initial symptoms include headache, palpitations, nausea, and vomiting, but arrhythmias and hypotension can occur, and fatal reactions have been recorded.

Alcoholic liver disease

In individuals with alcohol-related liver damage, drug disposal is diminished for a number of reasons. Circulating concentrations of drugs increase, with the result that the clinical effects might be exaggerated giving the impression of undue sensitivity (*Table 14*). Thus, first pass metabolism – the initial presentation of the drug to the liver – may be reduced by shunting of blood and 'sick' liver cells. Lessened availability of plasma proteins for drug binding allows more of the free drug to be delivered to the tissues, and distribution is affected by factors such as wasting, ascites, and diuretic treatment. There is some evidence[1] that cerebral sensitivity is increased in patients with chronic liver disease.

Table 14 *Liver damage*

Decreased drug breakdown causing increased drug activity	
barbiturates	isoniazid
benzodiazepines	propanolol
chlormethaziole	theophylline
opiates	frusemide
ampicillin	tolbutamide
rifampicin	phenytoin

Drugs with a substantial first pass metabolism are therefore dangerous in liver disease and doses need to be reduced accordingly; otherwise drugs whose extraction by the liver is limited or which are eliminated by the kidneys should be substituted.[5]

References

1. Hoyumpa, A.M.Jr and Schenker, S. (1982) Major Drug Interactions: Effects of Liver Disease, Alcohol, and Malnutrition. *Annual Review of Medicine* 33: 113–49.
2. Leading article (1980) Drugs and Alcohol. *British Medical Journal* 280: 507–08.
3. Linnoila, M., Mattila, M.J., and Kitchell, B.S. (1979) Drug Interactions with Alcohol. *Drugs* 18: 299–311.
4. Petrine, J., Stolz, A., and Kaplowitz, N. (1984) Drug Metabolism and Drug-Induced Liver Injury. In G. Gitnick (ed.) *Current Hepatology, Vol 4.* New York: John Wiley, pp. 247–312.
5. Williams, R.L. (1983) Drug Administration in Hepatic Disease. *New England Journal of Medicine* 309: 1616–622.

INDEX